POZ at 25

Empowering the HIV Community Since 1994

SMART+STRONG

New York

ISBN 978-0-578-60789-4

Published by Smart + Strong, POZ magazine chronicles the HIV/AIDS epidemic. Go to POZ.com for more information.

Printed in the United States of America

Smart + Strong
212 West 35th Street, 8th Floor
New York, NY 10001

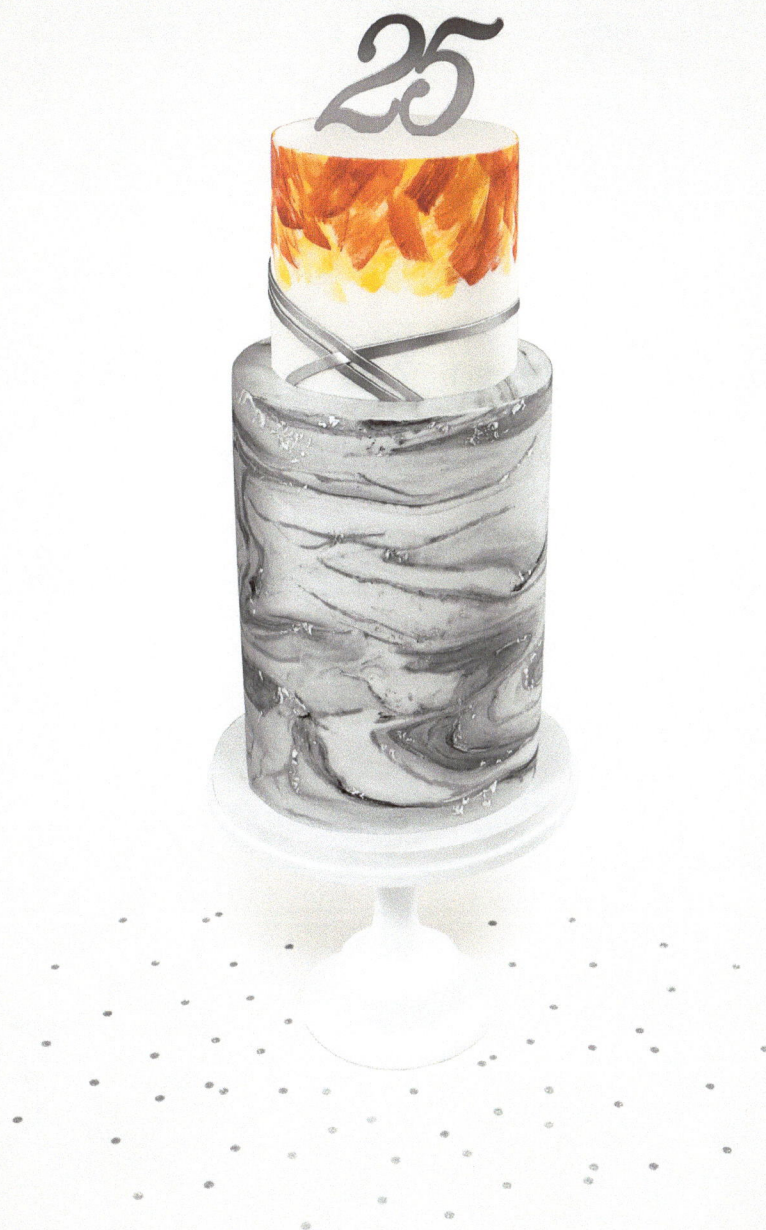

POZ has supported, looked after, championed, held up, informed and inspired for **25 years strong**. Thank you for everything you've done and all you continue to do. It's a privilege to commemorate this milestone with you. **Congratulations!**

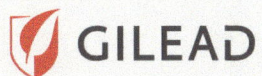

This book is dedicated to all POZ readers—past, present and future.
We remember those we've lost and uplift those who survive.
Thank you for your support.

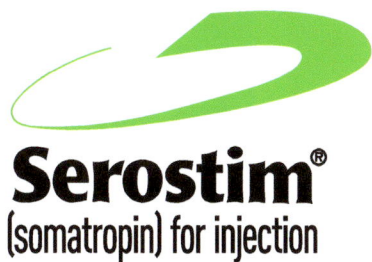

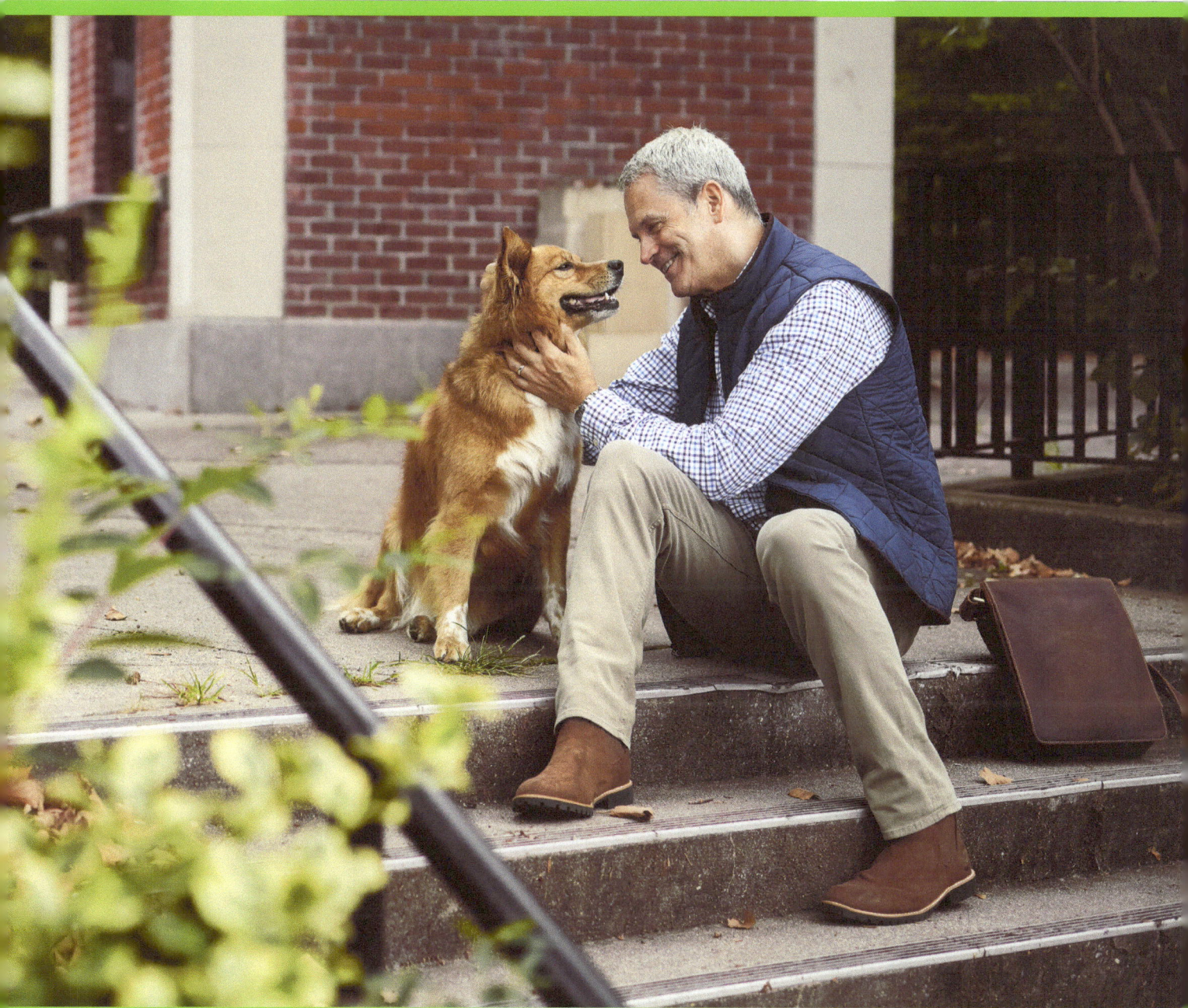

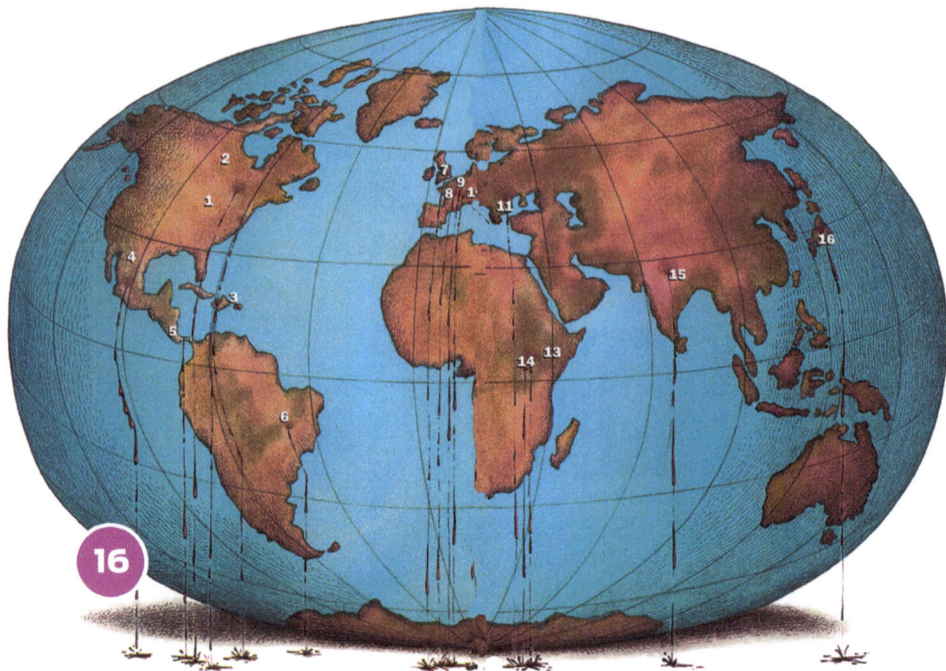

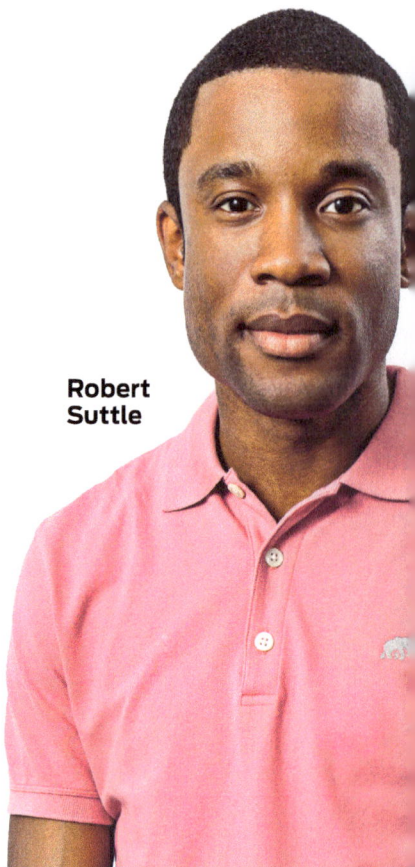

Robert Suttle

CONTENTS

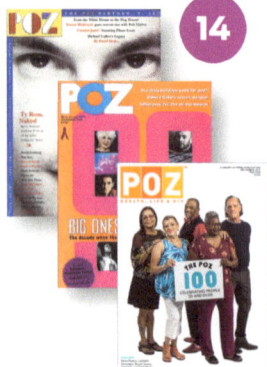

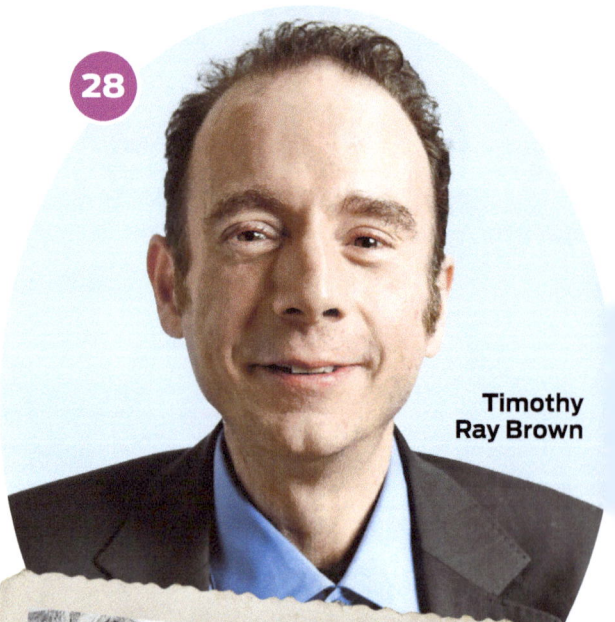

Timothy Ray Brown

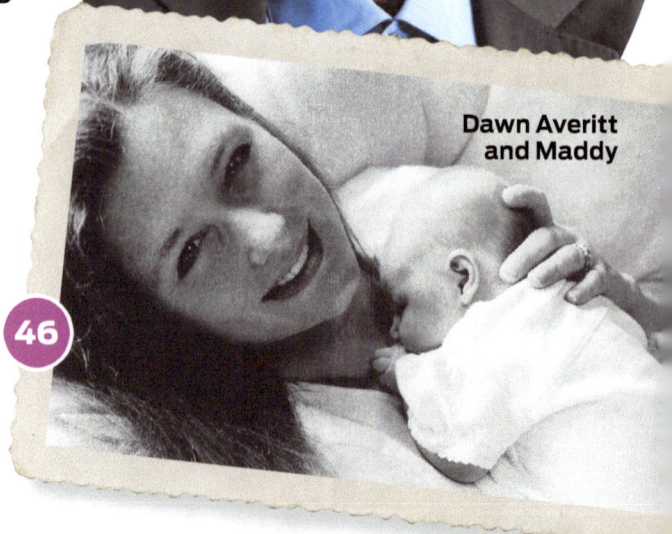

Dawn Averitt and Maddy

Bowman uses poetry, advocacy and music to speak up about HIV.

BASED ON
Her True Story

MUSIC AND ACTION IN THE POETRY OF MARY BOWMAN

BY CASEY HALTER
PHOTOGRAPHY BY JONATHAN TIMMES

IT HAS BEEN FIVE YEARS SINCE MARY BOWMAN first took the mic and disclosed her biggest secret to a live audience—she was born with HIV 26 years ago, in a Maryland suburb outside of Washington, DC, to a drug-addicted mother who died when Bowman was just 3 years old.

"The sickness she denied lies in my blood with a lesser value," is the big reveal in her poem "Dandelions," the first work she performed that declared her fears about dealing with her HIV status growing up.

Since Bowman's award-winning poetry collection, *LOTUS*, was published in 2011, the poet and songwriter has been at the forefront of a growing movement that uses storytelling and art to educate others about HIV/AIDS and to destroy the related stigma that can be as deadly as the virus itself.

Between recording her first R&B album, hosting monthly poetry open mics across the DC area and teaching her creative craft to local kids, Bowman has performed her poetry at HIV events and at colleges across the East Coast. In this edited POZ interview, the artist reflects on her accomplishments and shares her plans for the future.

Go to **poz.com/digital** to view the entire 25-year archive of POZ magazine—exactly as it appears in print!

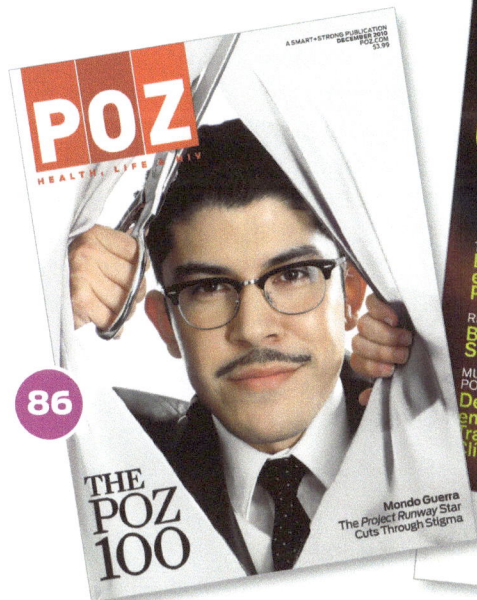

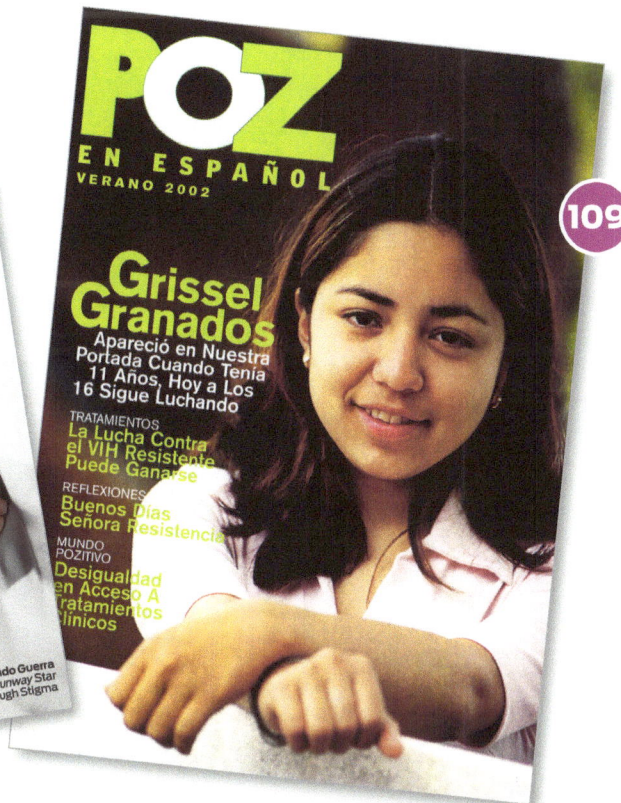

FOREWORD

WHEN THE FIRST ISSUE OF POZ WAS PUBLISHED IN 1994, ALL OF US INVOLVED KNEW WE HAD created a home in print (and, later, in pixels) for an important community voice that had the potential to change the course of the HIV epidemic and the lives of our readers.

We were proud of the beauty of its art and design, the audacity and ambition of our advocacy journalism and our commitment not only to speak truth to power but also to speak truth—often difficult truths—to one another and to the community.

We sought to model self-empowerment ideals, not just in the pursuit of our right to health care but also in the fight for our right to our sexuality, quality of life and dignity. In those early years especially, POZ gave voice to the different acute emotional responses of people living with HIV (PLHIV) to the protease and post-protease moments, the "Lazarus effect" and survivor's guilt.

We championed the project of rebuilding our lives and movement amid massive personal and generational trauma that persists to this day. We did this while enduring constant heartbreak as people who were central to POZ's early voice and unique identity, including Stephen Gendin, Jeffrey Schaire, Michael Callen, Pedro Zamora, Ilka Tanya Payán, David Feinberg, Kiki Mason, LeRoy Whitfield and so many others, were dying all around us.

The key to POZ's success has always been that our readers trust what they read in POZ more so than information they get from HIV/AIDS organizations, other media, the government, drug companies and even their own families and personal doctors. Speaking and listening to one another is what launched the PLHIV self-empowerment movement in the early '80s, a movement to which POZ is the journalistic heir.

I certainly never thought POZ would reach a quarter-century milestone, let alone that I would be here to witness it. But the occasion provides an opportunity to consider the activist context that led to the creation of the magazine. Many of us most responsible for POZ's legacy, including myself, Stephen Gendin and longtime editor-in-chief Walter Armstrong, were part of ACT UP, whose spectacular street theater, angry demonstrations and sophisticated advocacy are what first come to mind for many when they think of 1980s AIDS activism.

As much as POZ reflected that cultural zeitgeist, it also was—and is—grounded in the PLHIV self-empowerment movement, which predated ACT UP's 1987 founding. In my view, that movement also was more radical and far-reaching, causing a ripple effect in patient self-empowerment that has influenced health care throughout the world. Like POZ's editorial mission, that earlier advocacy centered on PLHIV, who looked toward one another for support and strength. Both prioritized connecting PLHIV with one another, creating power and change by building community.

In the early 1980s, the existing health care and social service delivery structure didn't serve people with AIDS, especially gay men, injection drug users, people of color, sex workers and poor people. We were left to die. Pioneering people with AIDS organized and wrote The Denver Principles manifesto (which codified ideals promoted by the women's health movement) to assert our right to a central role in the decision-making that so profoundly affected our lives. We created a parallel health care system of AIDS service organizations. There were no approved treatments, so we created buyers clubs to produce our own or to smuggle promising drugs from other countries. Research was slow or nonexistent, so we organized community clinicians to collect data from their patients through a community clinical trials network. With the PWA Newsline, the People With AIDS Coalition in New York pioneered our own media.

CONTINUED ▶

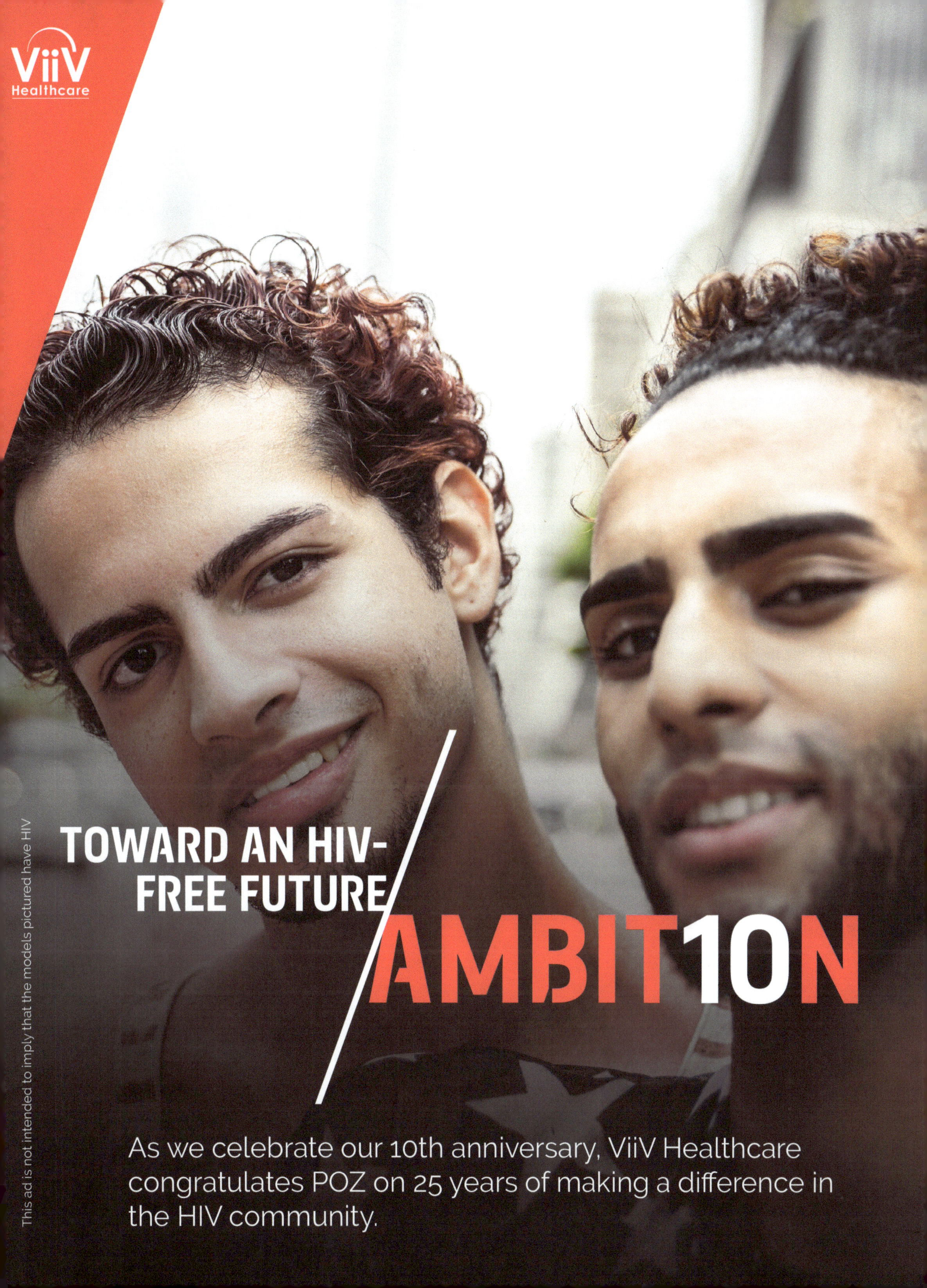

ViiV Healthcare
TOWARD AN HIV-FREE FUTURE
AMBIT10N
As we celebrate our 10th anniversary, ViiV Healthcare congratulates POZ on 25 years of making a difference in the HIV community.
This ad is not intended to imply that the models pictured have HIV

ACT UP activism was boisterous and demanding, driven in no small measure by white male privilege and mostly focused externally on the institutions of power, rather than the self-empowerment movement's internal focus on other PLHIV. ACT UP challenged the White House, Congress, the National Institutes of Health, the Food and Drug Administration, the media, pharmaceutical companies and others, successfully overhauling drug development and approval processes and expediting access to effective treatment.

Yet when drug development became the advocacy priority in the late '80s and early '90s, the feminist-inspired self-empowerment grassroots advocacy that preceded ACT UP began to fade from prominence within the AIDS movement. Getting PLHIV together with one another to provide peer support, develop our own strategies and speak with collective voices wasn't a priority for the emerging AIDS Inc. infrastructure.

Support for PLHIV networks declined as effective treatment was introduced in the mid-'90s, when POZ started. The community-created peer-to-peer service delivery system we developed moved incrementally toward the more dominant "benefactor/victim" service delivery paradigm.

By the late '90s, PLHIV began to be seen less as whole people deserving of support and sympathy and instead, through an increasingly racist lens, as an inherently dangerous population that posed a threat to society and needed to be monitored and controlled. Newly diagnosed PLHIV today are more isolated than in the early years, and HIV stigma is worse than ever, something most people who don't have HIV find startling.

Fortunately, PLHIV are responding as we did in those earliest days, organizing with our closest allies to create a flourishing PLHIV self-empowerment movement. New and growing PLHIV networks have brought us together to define our own agendas, to select and hold accountable leadership of our own choosing and to speak with collective voices.

Today, we are fighting far more than a virus. We are carrying forth the mandate issued by Vito Russo in 1990 when he declared "after we kick the shit out of this disease," we're going to "kick the shit out of this system, so that this never happens again." I am proud that POZ continues to be at our side in this epic struggle upon which so many lives depend.

Sean Strub
Founder, POZ

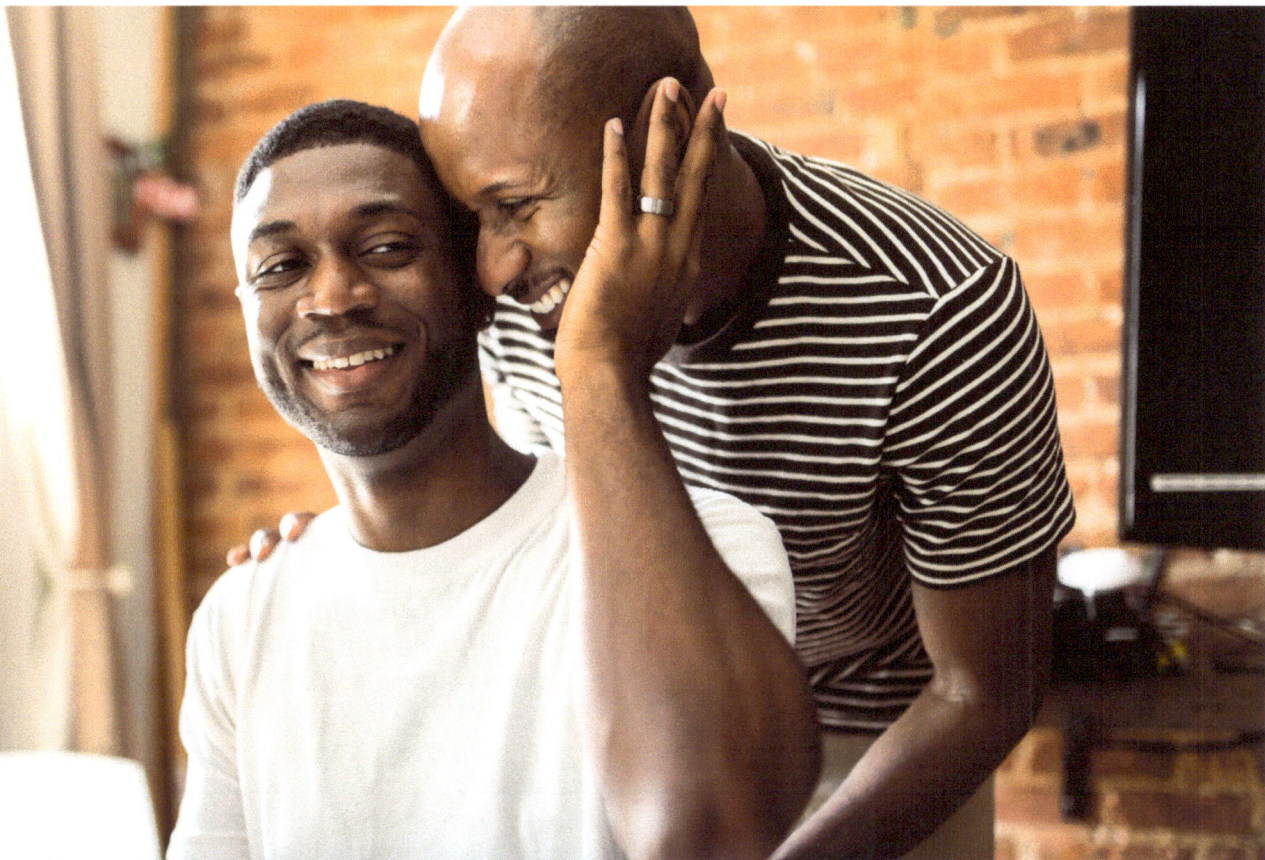

We're inspired
by Patients.

At Janssen, we're dedicated to addressing and solving some of the most important unmet medical needs of our time – in HIV and other areas. Driven by our commitment to patients, we develop innovative products, services and healthcare solutions to help people throughout the world.

We are Janssen. Our mission drives us. Patients inspire us. We collaborate with the world for the health of everyone in it.

Learn more at www.janssen.com

Janssen Infectious Diseases

PHARMACEUTICAL COMPANIES OF *Johnson&Johnson*

INTRODUCTION

I WILL ALWAYS REMEMBER THE DAY I WAS TOLD I HAVE HIV. IN 1992, THE DAY AFTER MY 22ND birthday, I was informed by my commanding officer in the United States Marine Corps Reserve that I had tested positive for the virus.

I sat and cried for a long time that day. Then I told my best friend, and we sat and cried together. The advent of effective HIV treatment in 1996 was still a dream when I tested positive. I never expected to see 30. The next few years only reinforced that dread as I lost loved ones to AIDS.

My experience is far from unique. The early '90s were trying times in the epidemic. The initial suffering of the '80s had been compounded by the continuing crisis—with no end in sight. It was a challenge to believe that tomorrow would be better.

POZ founder Sean Strub thought otherwise. Frustrated by the media's coverage of the AIDS epidemic, he launched the magazine in 1994 to amplify the voices of people living with HIV. Sean, who tested HIV positive in 1985, sold his life insurance policies to invest everything he had into the launch.

As Sean tells it in *Body Counts*, his 2014 memoir, "We tried to tell the story of the epidemic in all its complexities, through the experience of those with HIV. And we would do so in an attractive, engaging and hopeful format. On glossy paper."

Twenty-five years later, POZ persists. We've seen the fight for effective treatment lead to the fight for expansion of access to that treatment. We've gone from countering the fear of people who have HIV to promoting the fact that being undetectable means not being able to transmit the virus sexually.

Through it all, the core of our mission has remained unchanged—to be a mirror for the HIV community. From cure research to celebrities, from treatment improvements to personal stories, our coverage reflects the journeys of all of us affected by the virus.

In that spirit, for our 25th anniversary book cover, we created a collage of people (as well as dogs, artwork, a Muppet and more) spotlighted on our covers through the years. Although it's not exhaustive, the image is representative of our content.

The book cover was inspired by the cover of our April/May 2019 print magazine. In that issue, we caught up with 25 advocates who were deeply affected by their appearance on the cover. That feature story is reprinted in this book. Whatever the outcomes, appearing in POZ marked a milestone for them in their lives.

I certainly know what POZ meant to me as a reader, well before I had the honor of being editor-in-chief. I don't recall exactly which cover I saw first, but I can say for sure that I was captivated by the Pedro Zamora cover. That was the third issue of the magazine. All our covers and issues up to our 25th anniversary are highlighted in this book.

We hope you enjoy this retrospective of 25 years of POZ, and we thank you for reading!

Oriol R. Gutierrez Jr.
Editor-in-Chief, POZ

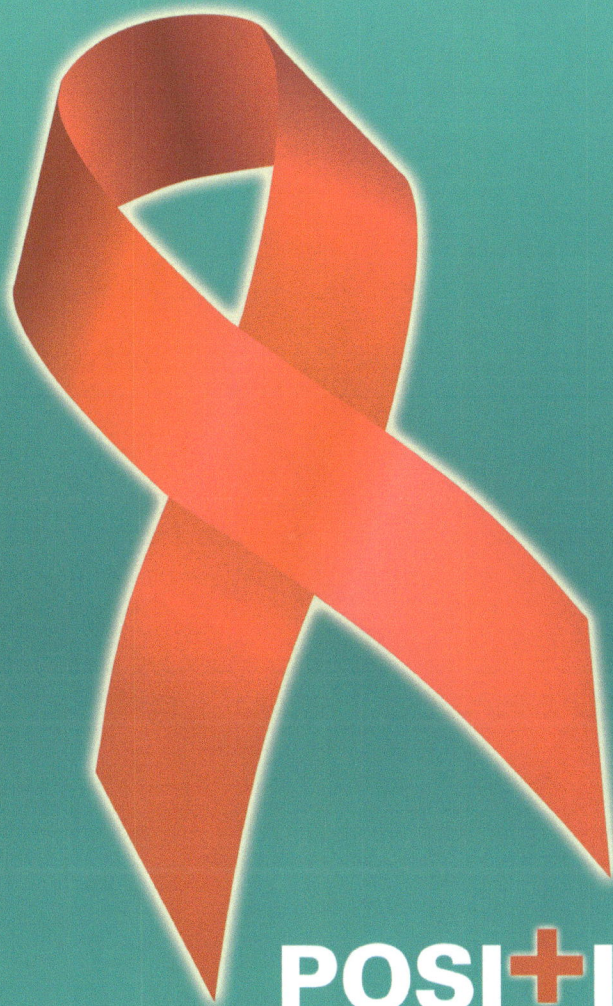

POSI✚IVELY COMMITTED

…together, for 30 years and counting

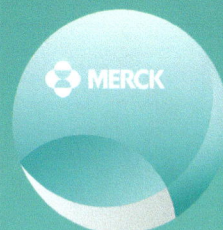

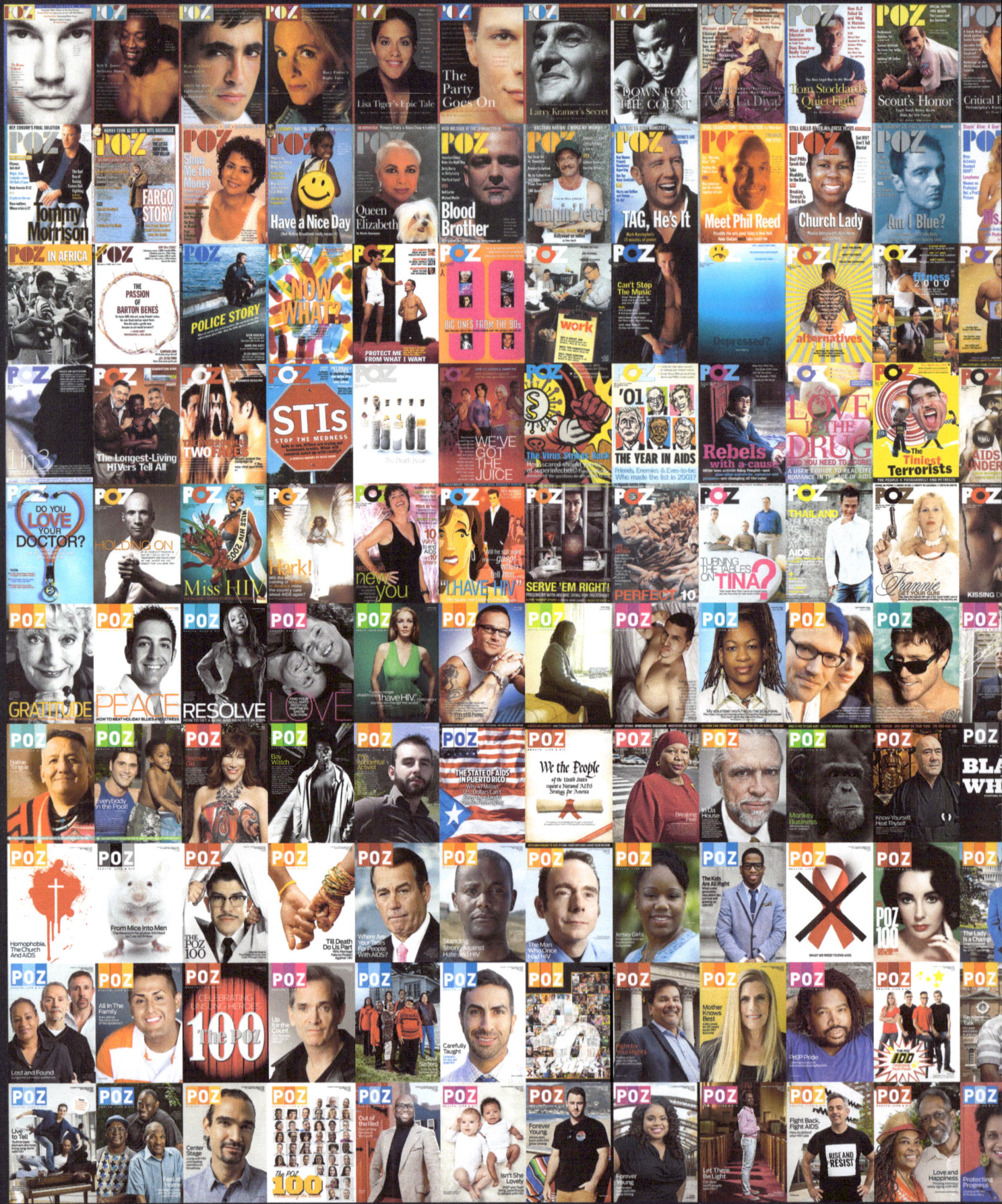

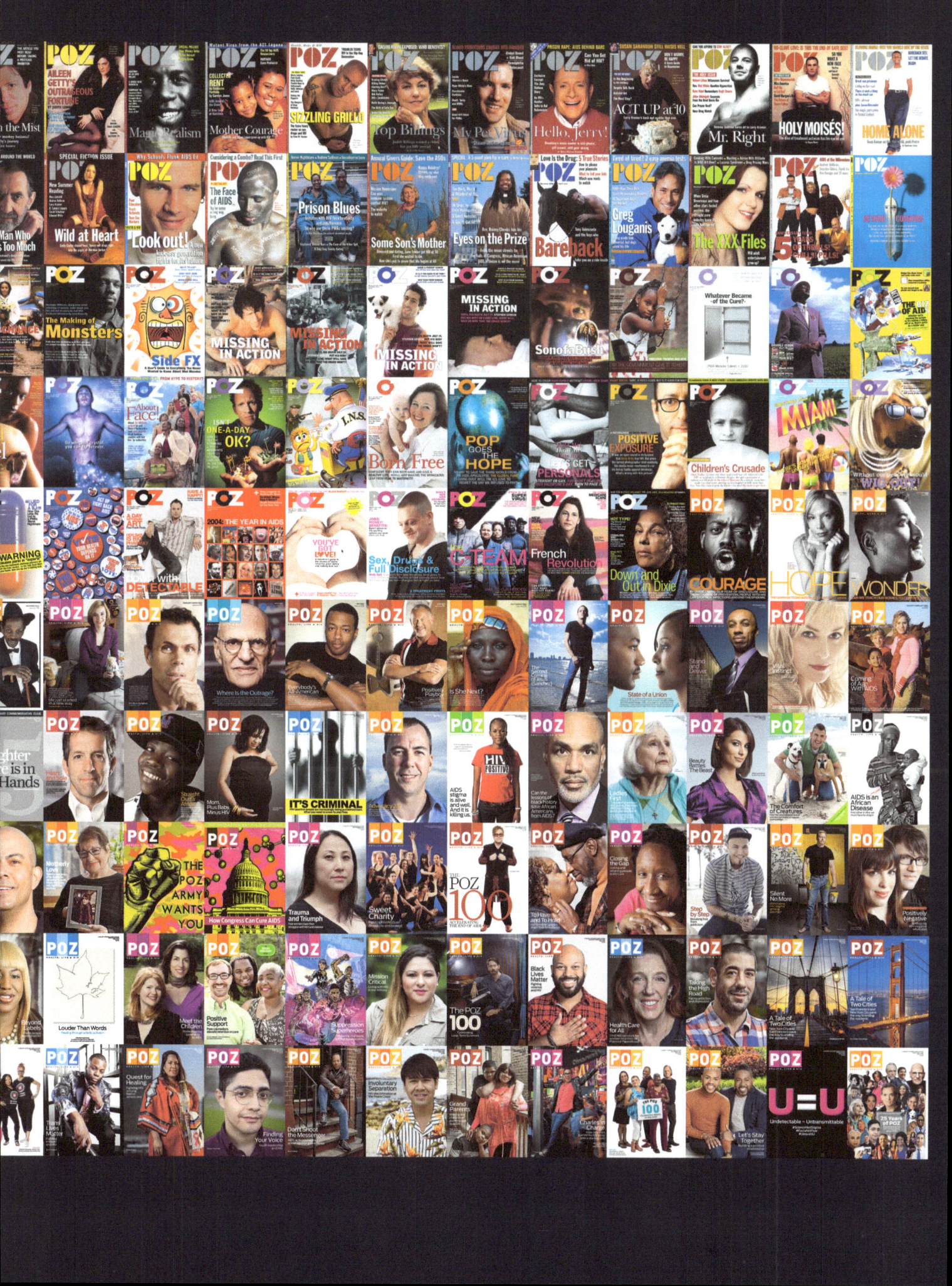

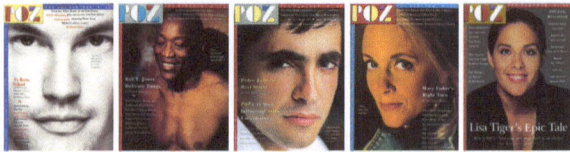

THE YEAR IN POZ

1994

April/May
(Premier Issue)

COVER: Ty Ross, the gay HIV-positive grandson of conservative icon Barry Goldwater. **INSIDE:** A stunning collection of black-and-white portraits of people living with AIDS by photographer Carolyn Jones (1). **PLUS:** An exclusive interview with activist and former Clinton administration aide Bob Hattoy, the first person living with AIDS to address a national convention (2).

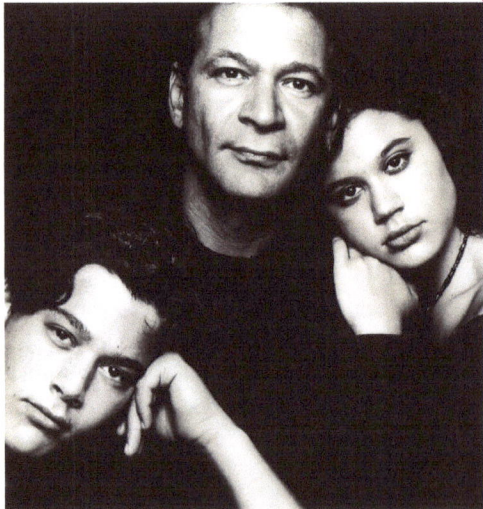

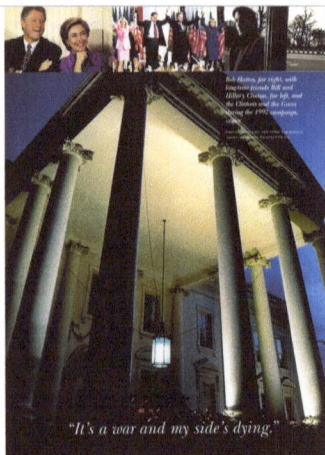

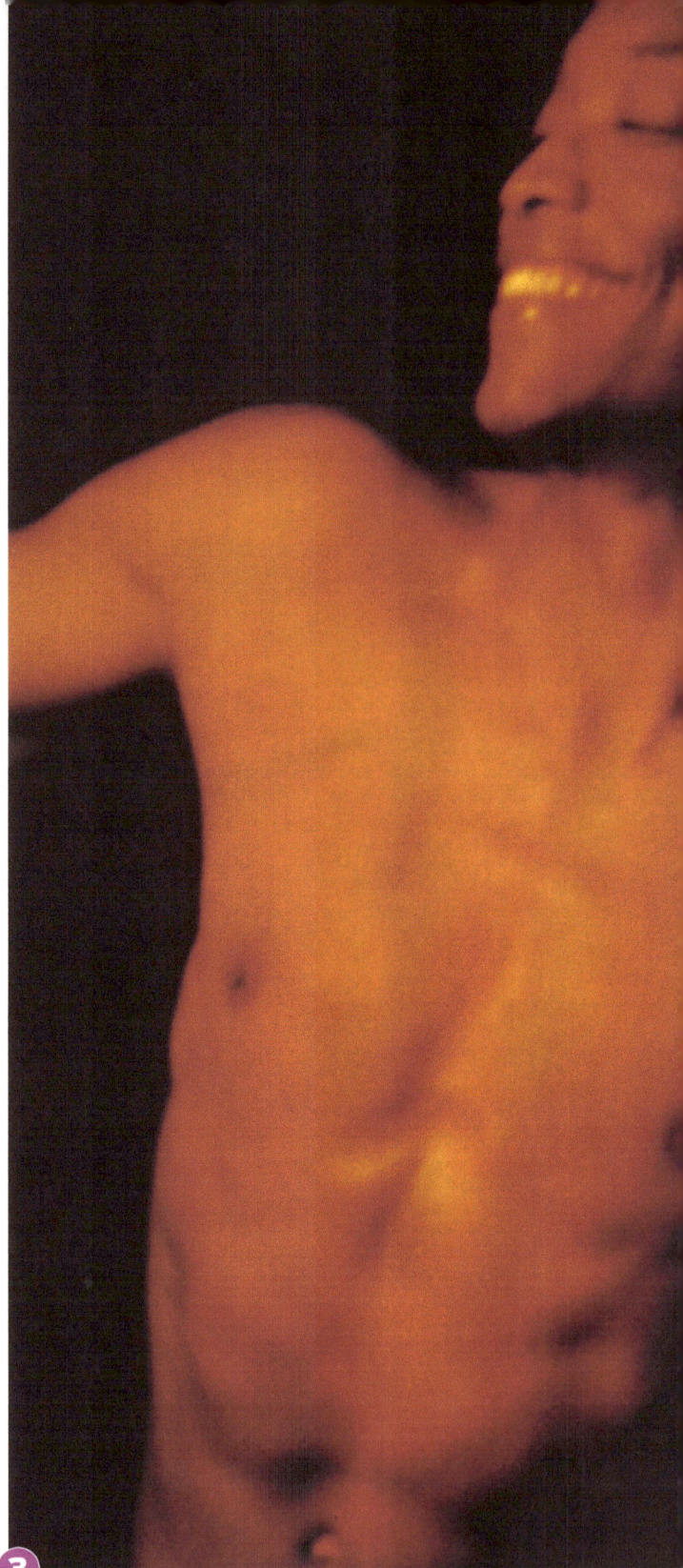

June/July

COVER: Dancer and choreographer Bill T. Jones (3). **INSIDE:** A look at the reemergence of tuberculosis as a public health threat; the hullabaloo about home HIV testing kits. **PLUS:** A tribute to Rudolf Nureyev, the greatest male ballet dancer of his generation.

August/September

COVER: HIV activist Pedro Zamora of MTV's *The Real World*. **INSIDE:** A portfolio of the illustrations of fashion artist Antonio López (4); an interview with comedian Joan Rivers; a feature on the use of anabolic steroids among people living with HIV. **PLUS:** POZ compiles a list of 50 influential AIDS policymakers.

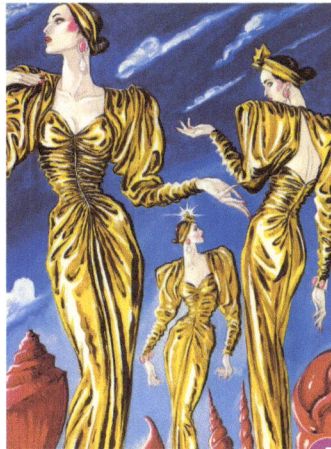

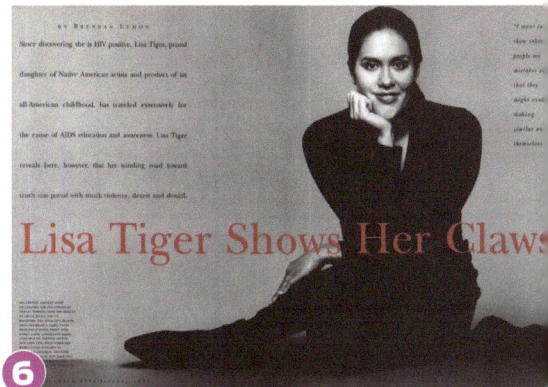

October/November

COVER: Mary Fisher, who rocked the Republican National Convention in 1992 with her eloquent calls for compassion toward people living with AIDS. **INSIDE:** A feature on AIDS and health care reform; an interview with Boy George, who speaks frankly about AIDS and pop music's persistent homophobia (5). **PLUS:** A test drive of the new female condom.

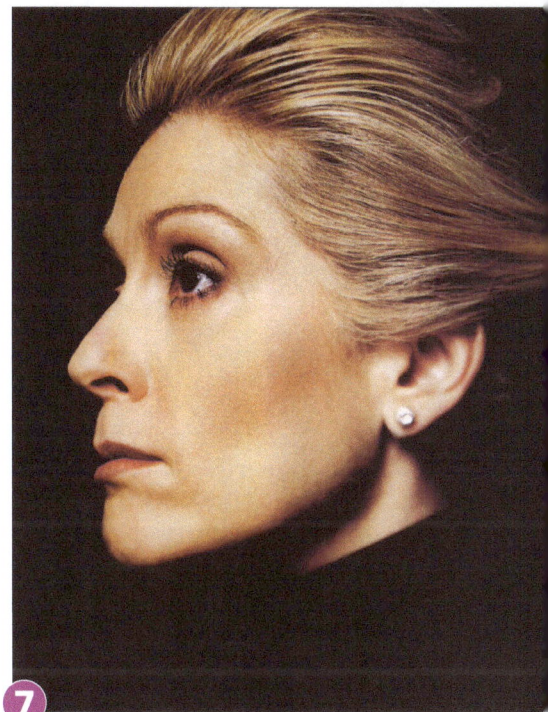

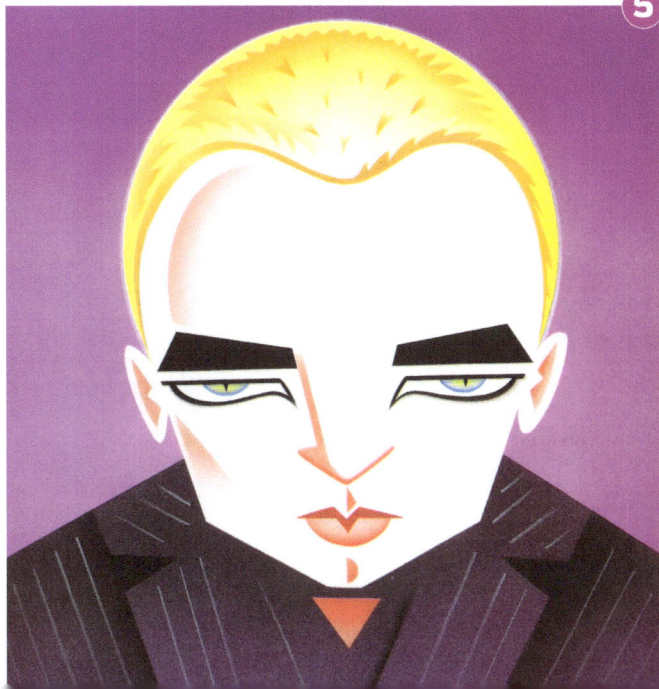

December/ January 1995

COVER: Native American activist Lisa Tiger (6). **INSIDE:** A look inside San Francisco's Cannabis Buyers Club; a feature delving into the AIDS funeral pickets organized by the Reverend Fred Phelps and the Westboro Baptist Church; POZ editor-in-chief Richard Pérez-Feria interviews actress, activist and ally Judith Light about her role in the fight (7). **PLUS:** A look at Hollywood's biggest AIDS moguls.

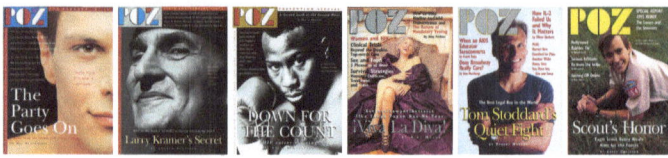

1995

Dancer from the Dance

BY HAL RUBENSTEIN

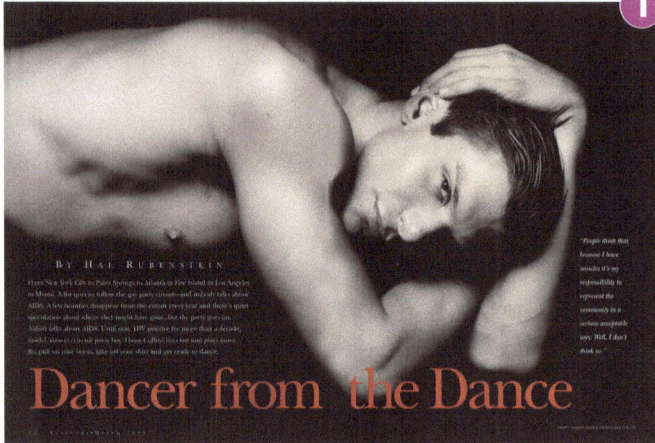

February/March

COVER: Thom Collins, an HIV-positive model and dancer, talks about AIDS on the gay party circuit (**1**). **INSIDE:** A look at how AIDS groups overcome fund-raising challenges (**2**); a giving guide to AIDS service organizations; true horror stories from AIDS fundraising galas. **PLUS:** Wilson Cruz of *My So-Called Life* on coming out in the era of AIDS.

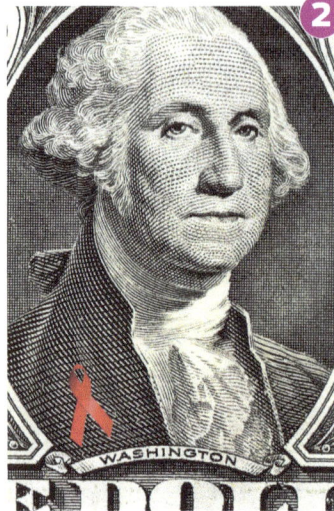

April/May

COVER: Larry Kramer ("the father of AIDS activism") makes his first cover appearance with an interview by pundit Andrew Sullivan. **INSIDE:** An excerpt from *Breaking the Surface*, a new memoir by Olympic medalist Greg Louganis (**3**); do you know what's in the water you're drinking? **PLUS:** ABC News anchor Peter Jennings discusses his HIV-related journalism (**4**).

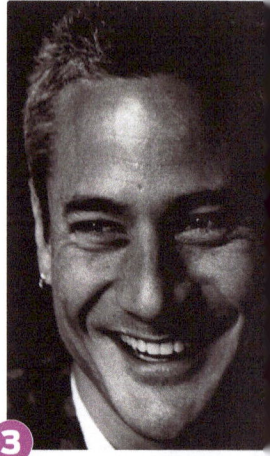

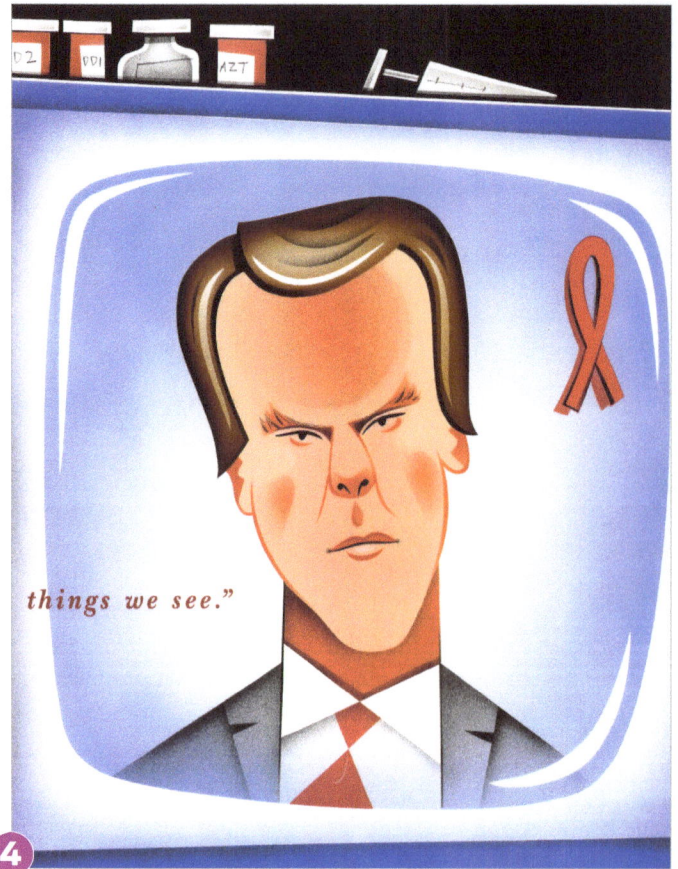

things we see."

June/July

COVER: Lamar "Kidfire" Parks, an HIV-positive boxer and formerly the world's No. 1 middleweight contender, talks about how the virus ended his career. **INSIDE:** HIV prevention activism moves to the forefront as safer sex is scrutinized. **PLUS:** Biotechnology companies pioneer new high-stakes HIV research; HIV-positive photographer John Dugdale on losing his sight to cytomegalovirus, or CMV (**5**).

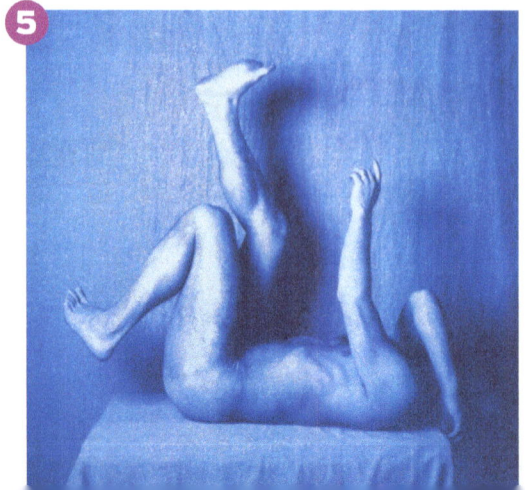

August/September

COVER: Actress-lawyer-activist Ilka Tanya Payán is a fighter with no fear. **INSIDE:** Spotlighting the needs of HIV-positive women that are not being addressed (**6**); why pregnancy is the one thing that makes policymakers interested in the lives of women with HIV. **PLUS:** Keeping pets and their HIV-positive owners together (**7**).

6

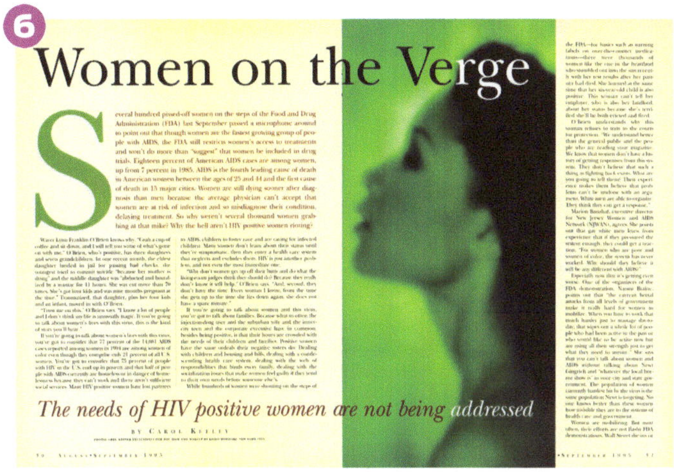

Women on the Verge

The needs of HIV positive women are not being addressed

BY CAROL KELLY

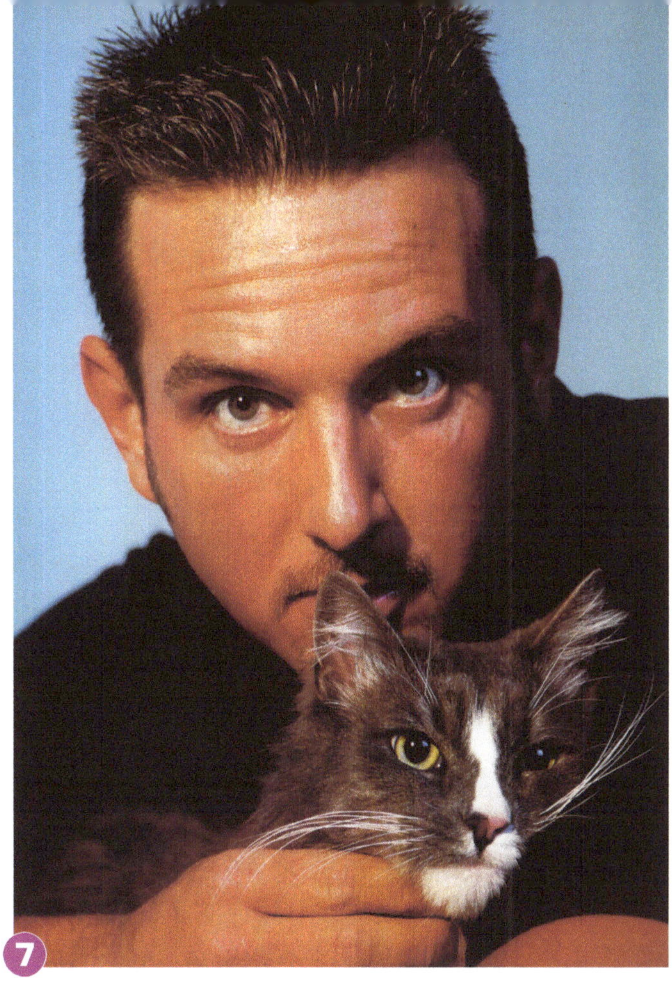

7

October/November

COVER: Public-interest lawyer Tom Stoddard fights AIDS discrimination loudly and his HIV quietly. **INSIDE:** The treatment known as IL-2 highlights the AIDS research turf war between virologists and immunologists (**8**); does Broadway really care about AIDS? **PLUS:** Political organizer and activist Rae Lewis-Thornton educates the Black community about HIV.

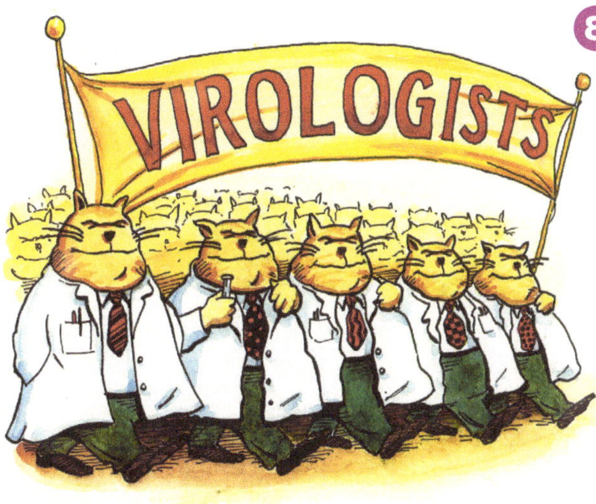

8

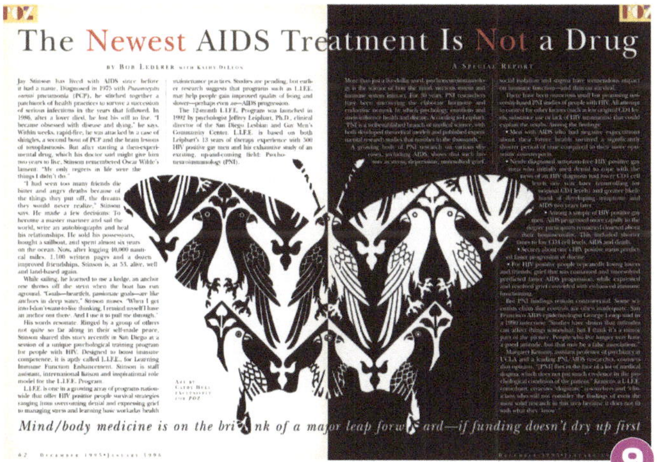

VIROLOGISTS

The Newest AIDS Treatment Is Not a Drug

BY BOB LEDERER WITH KATHI DELUCA

A SPECIAL REPORT

Mind/body medicine is on the brink of a major leap forward—if funding doesn't dry up first

9

December/January 1996

COVER: Henry Nicols—Cooperstown's most famous Eagle Scout—is all grown up with many places to go. **INSIDE:** A retrospective of the sublime, the ridiculous and the heroic events of the past year; Tinseltown's script about AIDS is good, but the picture is not always pretty. **PLUS:** The newest AIDS treatment is not a drug (**9**).

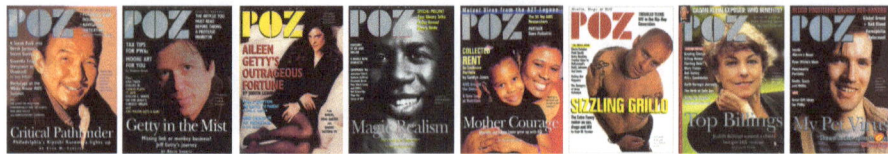

THE YEAR IN POZ

1996

May

COVER: Heiress Aileen Getty is used to being defined by the people around her—but now, she's making her own mark. **INSIDE:** A surreal vision through the black-and-white lens of Steven Arnold (**3**); the FDA approves new antiretrovirals in record time. **PLUS:** *The Young and the Restless* pushes the AIDS envelope firmly but softly.

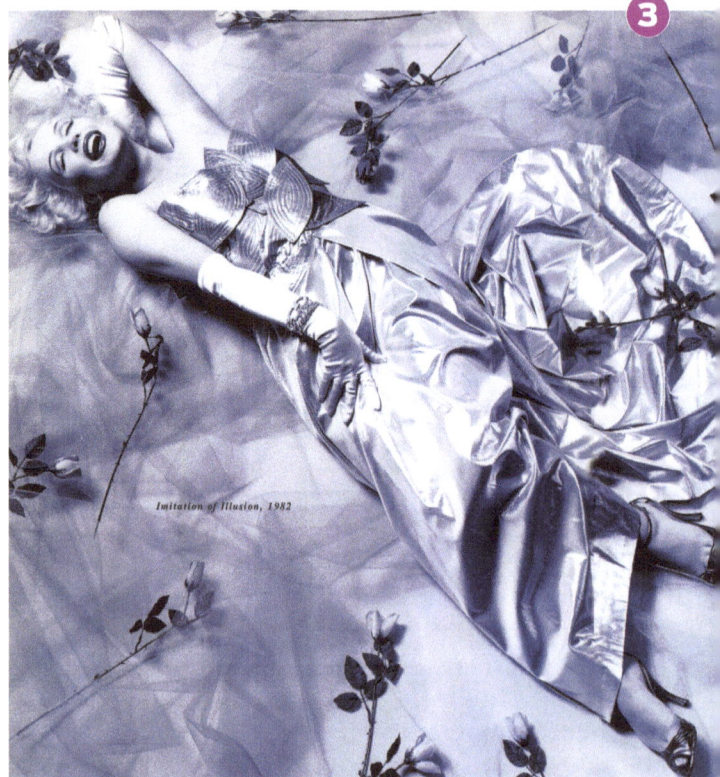

Imitation of Illusion, 1982

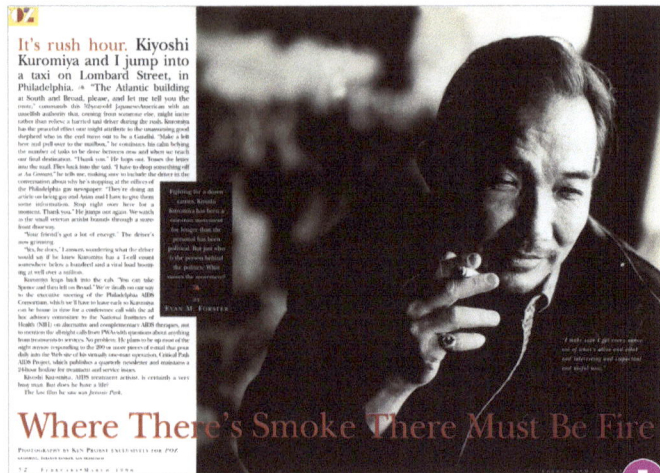

Where There's Smoke There Must Be Fire

February/March

COVER: Fighting for a dozen causes, Kiyoshi Kuromiya is a one-man movement (**1**). **INSIDE:** Community-based AIDS research is both sparking answers and raising eyebrows; trading life insurance for cash doesn't have to be hard, but may the seller beware. **PLUS:** *Seinfeld* mixes messages on contraceptives and AIDS and comes up with unprotected sex.

April

COVER: Jeff Getty receives a transplant of baboon bone marrow cells as an experimental procedure to treat his HIV (**2**). **INSIDE:** Frank Moore's art blends nature and medicine; U.S. military to give people with HIV the boot. **PLUS:** The article you must read before taking a protease inhibitor.

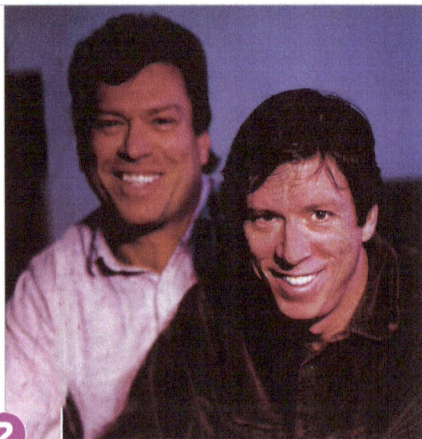

June/July

COVER: Magic Johnson may not want to talk about HIV, but he has forever changed the way America sees people living with the virus. **INSIDE:** Our annual report card on AIDS service organizations; preplanning, expert care and human compassion can help manage the trauma of dementia. **PLUS:** Acupuncture stimulates the body to rebuild its healing ability (**4**).

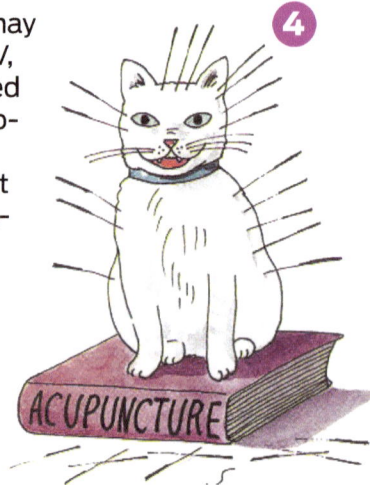

ACUPUNCTURE

August/September

COVER: Michelle Lopez (with daughter Raven) has seen the dark side—now she's spreading the light. **INSIDE:** The 50 top AIDS researchers; *Rent* is this season's hottest ticket on Broadway, and it's giving people with HIV a new lease on love. **PLUS:** How antiretroviral drugs may backfire through mutations (5).

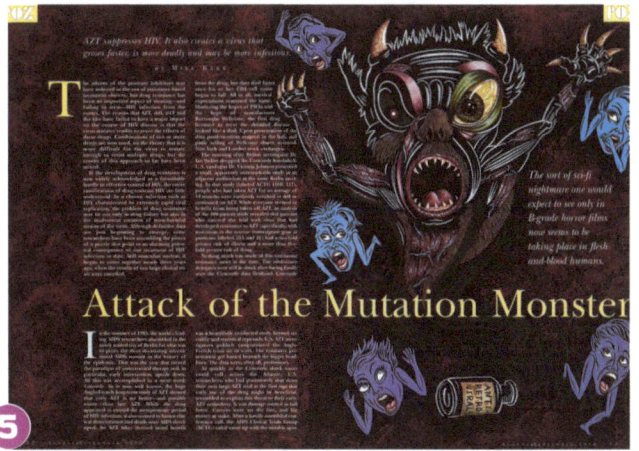

Attack of the Mutation Monster

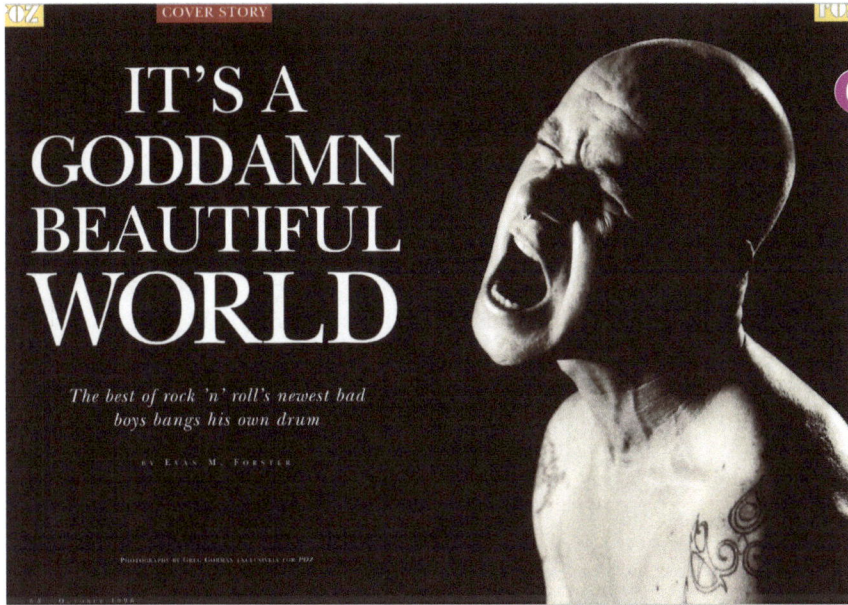

October

COVER: Rocker Brian Grillo bangs to his own drum (6). **INSIDE:** The American Medical Association endorses mandatory HIV testing for pregnant women; five new CDs chronicle the epidemic in song. **PLUS:** Transgender diva Alexandra Billings on disclosing her HIV-positive status (7).

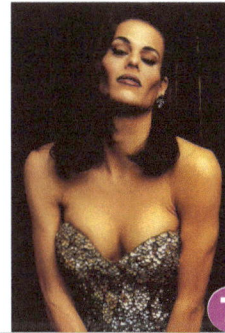

November

COVER: Outspoken public servant Judith Billings wears her politics on her lapel (8). **INSIDE:** Pundits on Election '96 and what it means for PWAs; politics are killing people who inject drugs. **PLUS:** An exclusive excerpt from the supremely dishy exposé, *Tarnished Sequins* by former AIDS Project Los Angeles board member Michael Anketell.

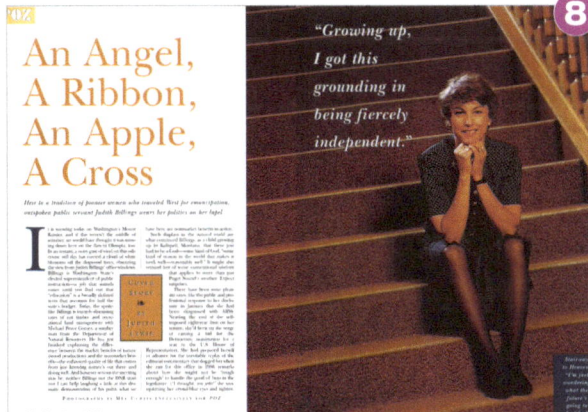

December/January 1997

COVER: Shawn Decker tested positive at the end of sixth grade. Nine years later, he's posting his story on the internet, becoming one of the first bloggers living with HIV. **INSIDE:** How people with hemophilia are fighting back; thanks to greed, corruption and cowardice, AIDS goes globe-trotting (9). **PLUS:** Artist Patrick Webb's adventures with Punchinello.

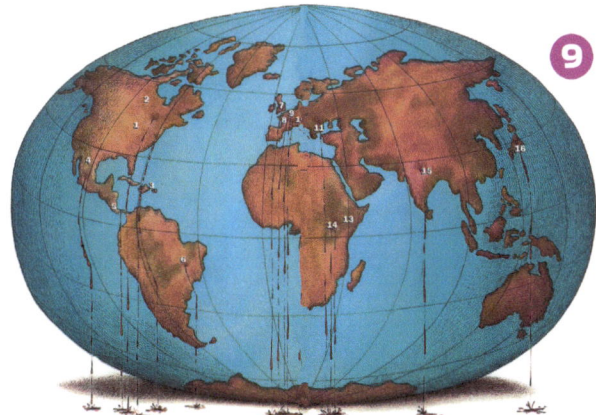

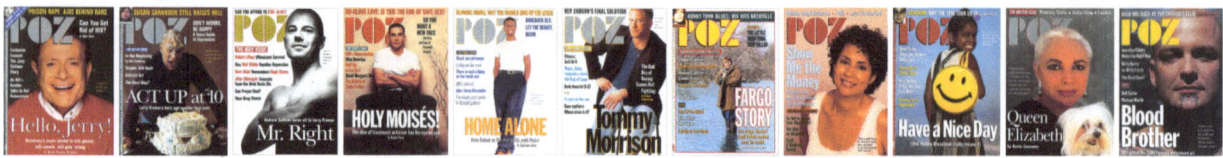

THE YEAR IN POZ

1997

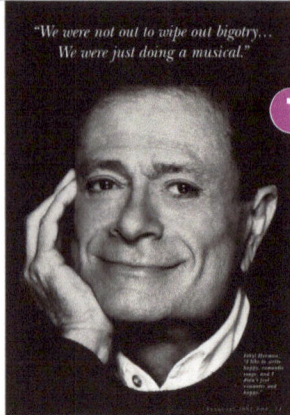

JERRY HERMAN was in typically ebullient spirits at the official first day of rehearsals for the latest revival of *Hello, Dolly!* No matter that Carol Channing was the star; the New York City press eagerly huddled around Herman as though he

"We were not out to wipe out bigotry... We were just doing a musical."

He Is What He Is

Showtune master Jerry Herman, the bard of Broadway, makes no apologies

February

COVER: Broadway tunesmith Jerry Herman wants the world to know about the new HIV treatments (**1**). **INSIDE:** How HIV is spread through the prison system; researchers touted the end of the epidemic at last year's International AIDS Conference in Vancouver, but will the new protease inhibitors work for everyone? **PLUS:** An interview with an HIV-positive sex worker.

March

COVER: On ACT UP's 10th anniversary, a name-calling essay by cofounder Larry Kramer, who writes, "Hope makes people lazy." **INSIDE:** An interview with actress and activist Susan Sarandon; a look at ACT UP's early roots (**2**). **PLUS:** An ad for the nationwide POZ Life Expo Tour, cohosted by the National Minority AIDS Council (NMAC).

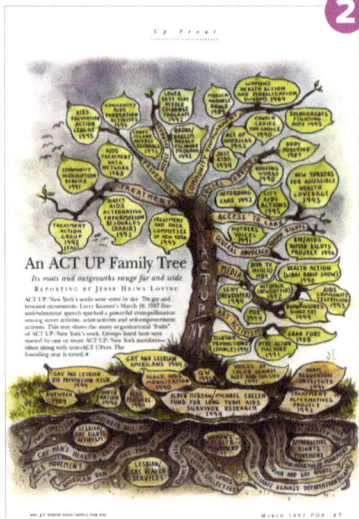

An ACT UP Family Tree
Its roots and outgrowths range far and wide

April

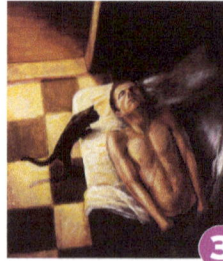

COVER: Larry Kramer interviews British import Andrew Sullivan, a controversial (and conservative) gay pundit and author. **INSIDE:** An exclusive excerpt from *After Midnight: The Life and Death of Brad Davis*, star of 1978's *Midnight Express* and 1985's *The Normal Heart*; an essay by the Reverend Dr. Mel White. **PLUS:** Gore Vidal reflects on the paintings of his late half-nephew Hugh Steers (**3**).

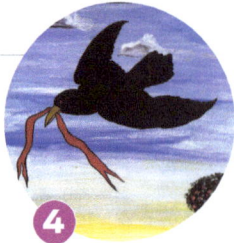

May

COVER: Life lessons from Moisés Agosto, treatment advocate for NMAC. **INSIDE:** More people with HIV are giving the old nip-and-tuck a try. **PLUS:** Fears of reinfection and sexually transmitted infections make HIV-positive couples think twice about ditching the condoms (**4**).

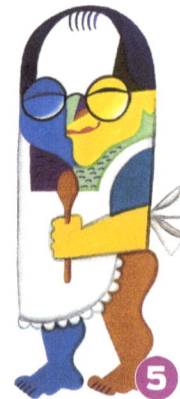

June

COVER: Sean Sasser on life after the loss of partner Pedro Zamora, star of MTV's *The Real World*. **INSIDE:** A Q&A with Jason Alexander (*Seinfeld*'s George Costanza), who's in the film version of *Love! Valour! Compassion!* (**5**). **PLUS:** An excerpt from Gabriel Rotello's *Sexual Ecology* asks whether gay men must choose between monogamy and extinction.

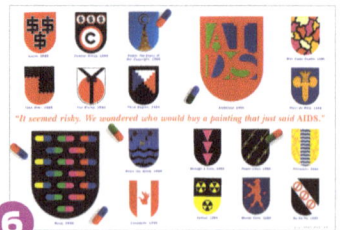

July

COVER: The Sports Issue profiles boxing champ Tommy Morrison, who has HIV but says the virus doesn't cause AIDS. **INSIDE:** A gallery of AIDS art by the Canadian collective General Idea (**6**). **PLUS:** A cure for cryptosporidium, a parasite that has been killing people with AIDS.

August

COVER: Cyndi Potete, the first North Dakotan ever charged with attempted murder by HIV. **INSIDE:** POZ goes to Nashville and finds that HIV in Music City is full of heartbreak and loneliness. **PLUS:** A portfolio of witty, wacky and wonderful theater costumes by the late Howard Crabtree (7).

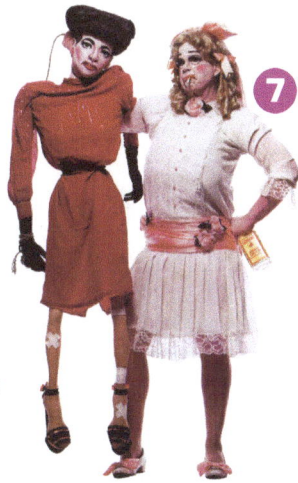

September

COVER: POZ spends a week with HIV-positive mom Susan Rodriguez as she navigates social services and finds that not working is a full-time job (8). **INSIDE:** Do protease-based treatments threaten the disability benefits of people with AIDS? **PLUS:** A gallery of Mary Berridge's photos of HIV-positive women.

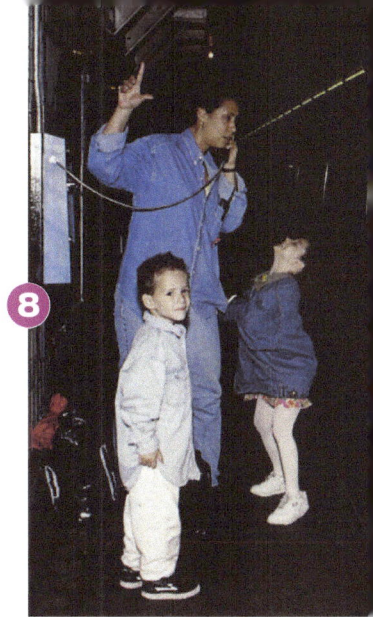

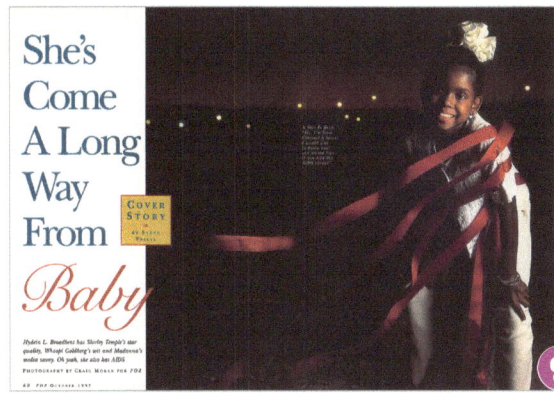

October

COVER: Born with HIV, 13-year-old Hydeia Broadbent, is a media-savvy AIDS advocate who spoke at the 1996 Republican National Convention (9). **INSIDE:** The mordant humor of *Diseased Pariah News,* an irreverent zine for and about people living with HIV. **PLUS:** Dan Savage on the (false) HIV-as-motive rumor behind Andrew Cunanan's murder of Gianni Versace and four others.

November

COVER: For the British Issue, Kevin Sessums interviews Elizabeth Taylor, patron saint of AIDS (10). **INSIDE:** Playwright Neil Bartlett explains why his AIDS oeuvre isn't about AIDS; a profile of author (and longtime survivor) Edmund White. **PLUS:** A letter from guest editor Aiden Shaw.

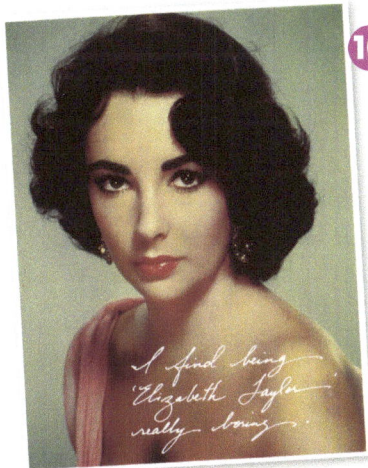

December

COVER: Artist Ron Athey, infamous for his body modifications, piercing performances and works involving blood (11). **INSIDE:** The legal battle faced by people with AIDS who use pot for medical purposes; a tribute to Diana, Princess of Wales. **PLUS:** ABC's annual HIV-themed special, *In a New Light,* ends after five years.

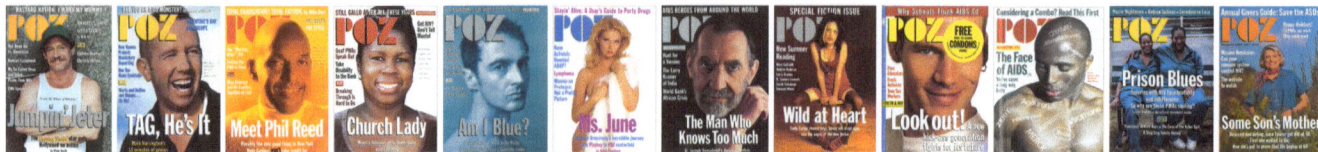

1998

January

COVER: Actor Michael Jeter on Tinseltown wannabes, media gossipmongers, gay moralists and his own troubled path to happiness. **INSIDE:** Adopted PWAs line up for the Terminal Illness Emergency Search, which helps adoptees find their birth parents; photographer Kire Godal looks at the big picture of AIDS in Kenya (**1**). **PLUS:** The first-ever organ transplant for people living with HIV.

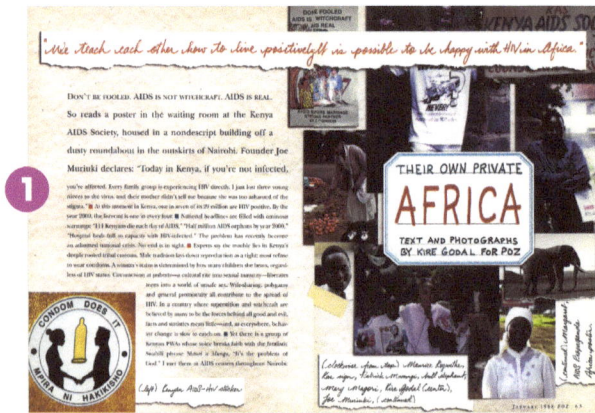

February

COVER: Treatment Action Group's Mark Harrington tells POZ what it means to have won a MacArthur "genius" grant (**2**). **INSIDE:** If you thought teenage acne was tough, HIV has an unsightly surprise in store for you; mandatory HIV name reporting is back, but this time the battle lines are redrawn. **PLUS:** A new exhibit showcases the work of downtown artist Jack Smith, who mixed mediums and metaphors.

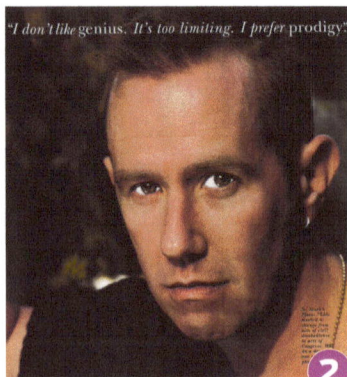

"I don't like genius. It's too limiting. I prefer prodigy."

March

COVER: New York City Councilman Phil Reed is openly gay, HIV positive and ready to fight for his constituents. **INSIDE:** Post-exposure prevention (PEP) is HIV's morning-after pill; remembering socialist-realist painter Patrick Angus and his art (**3**). **PLUS:** International Mr. Leather 1996 flaunts his family values.

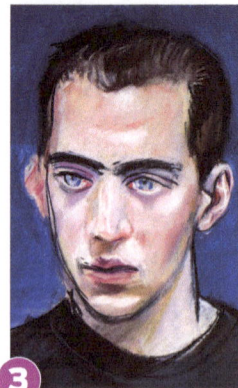

April

COVER: Monica Johnson turns God's country into AIDS country in rural Louisiana. **INSIDE:** HIV education is lost in translation for the deaf; AIDS trailblazer Robert Gallo, MD, shares new strategies and a few surprises (**4**). **PLUS:** Richard Renaldi photographs the West Village waterfront in his new series, *Pier 45*.

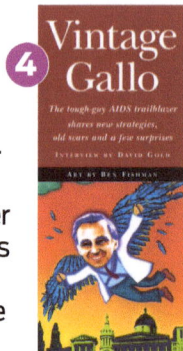

May

COVER: Performance artist John Kelly describes how he includes AIDS in his work. **INSIDE:** A roundtable on HIV criminalization; people with HIV are adding a dash of herbs to their treatment stews (**5**). **PLUS:** Choreographer Mark Dendy whips up a healthy brew of spirituality and skepticism.

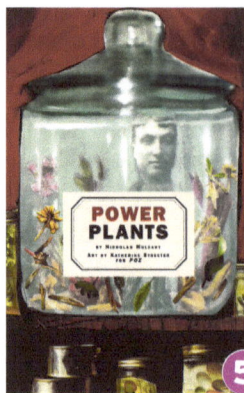

June

COVER: Former Playboy centerfold Rebekka Armstrong is talking up safe sex at Catholic schools and posing for POZ (**6**). **INSIDE:** A tactical alliance between drug companies and AIDS advocates is bankrupting drug assistance programs nationwide. **PLUS:** How to take the tumors and treatments in stride.

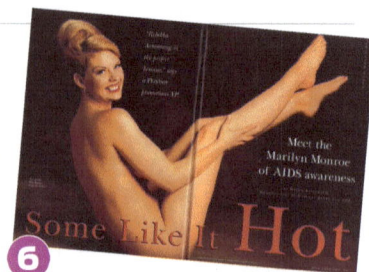

July

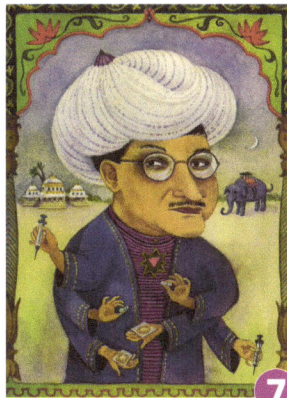

COVER: Joseph Sonnabend, MD, has been at the forefront of the AIDS epidemic, helping to create one of the first publications on safer sex and cofounding the organization that would become amfAR. **INSIDE:** Ashok Row Kavi is the Larry Kramer of India (**7**); the World Bank's African crisis is killing people living with HIV/AIDS; reinvigorating the national effort for vaccine research. **PLUS:** Secrets and lies about your HIV medications.

August

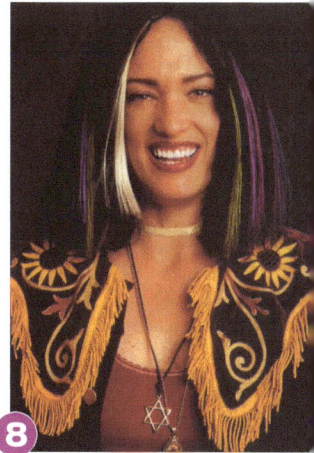

COVER: Emily Carter took a dark journey, but now, she's one of her generation's brightest writers (**8**). **INSIDE:** New fiction by seven of our favorite authors; performance artist Karen Finley wants you to remember those we lost to AIDS. **PLUS:** Miss America Kate Shindle dares to talk to students across the nation about HIV prevention despite some restrictions on what she can say.

September

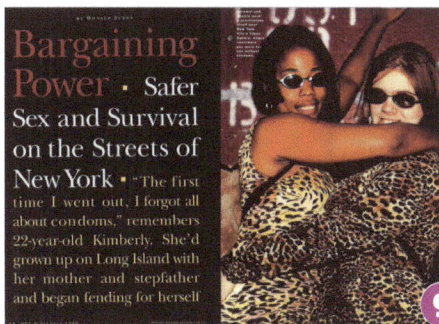

COVER: Eight HIV-positive youth discuss the virus and its effect on their generation. **INSIDE:** Why HIV education is failing America's teens; hepatitis C suddenly has people with HIV talking, testing and treating; safer sex and survival on the streets of New York City (**9**). **PLUS:** Meet Heather Farkas, a 17-year-old prep school prevention expert.

October

COVER: The art of selling HIV drugs, featuring model Michael Weathers (**10**). **INSIDE:** The aftermath of Sean Strub's drug holiday; the latest on early drug intervention; Dan Pallotta's fabled bike rides raise millions for AIDS, but is it time to look a gift horse in the mouth? **PLUS:** A recap of the 12th International AIDS Conference in Geneva.

November

COVER: Against all odds, inmates have emerged as their own best AIDS educators and advocates. **INSIDE:** The children of an inmate living with AIDS hold their family together; how treatment and care for inmates living with HIV varies dramatically from prison to prison (**11**). **PLUS:** Mark Tucker beats the odds behind bars.

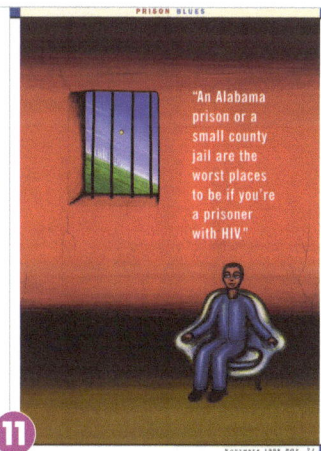

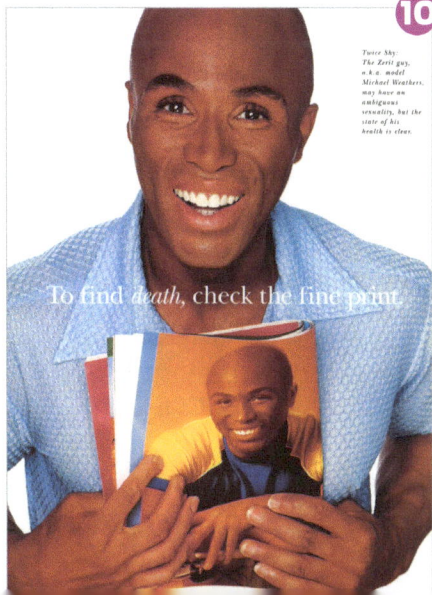

December

COVER: Jane Fowler is one of many people aging with HIV who are considering safer sex as part of their retirement plan. **INSIDE:** POZ's Annual Givers Guide; Sri Lanka wakes up late to AIDS; the public life of artist Felix Gonzalez-Torres. **PLUS:** If HIV meds can't completely rid the body of the virus, can the immune system contain what HIV is left (**12**)?

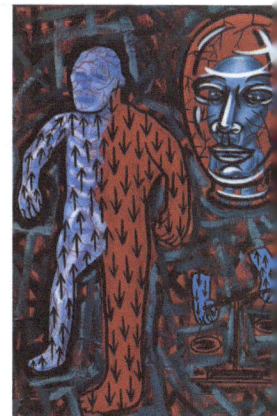

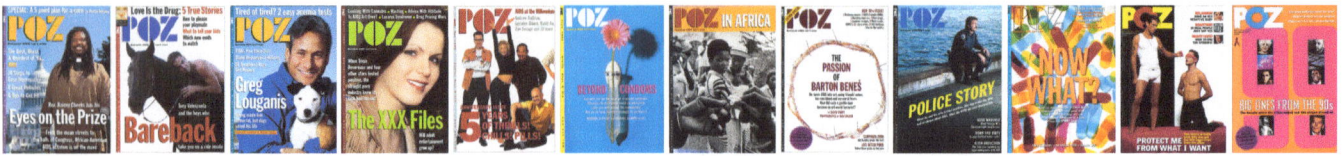

1999

January

COVER: A profile of the Reverend Rainey Cheeks, founder of Us Helping Us, Washington, DC's first AIDS service organization for gay Black men (1). **INSIDE:** The best, worst and weirdest news from 1998; how African-American leaders are tackling the epidemic in their midst; 10 steps to ease peripheral neuropathy. **PLUS:** Mario Cooper interviews San Francisco Mayor Willie Brown about his record on HIV/AIDS.

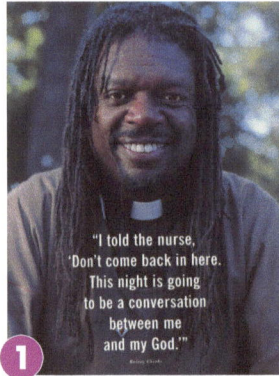

"I told the nurse, 'Don't come back in here. This night is going to be a conversation between me and my God.'"

— Rainey Cheeks

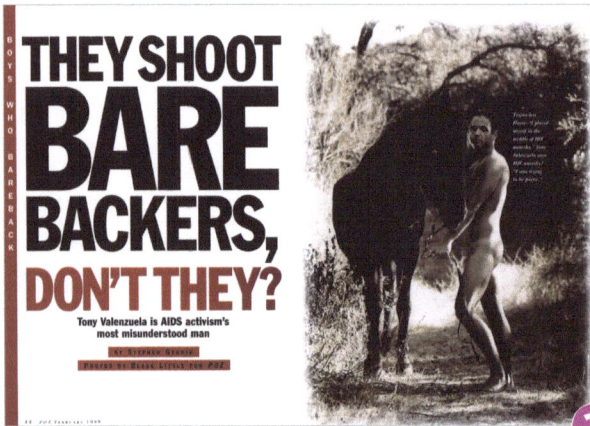

February

COVER: Tony Valenzuela talks about barebacking and how he became AIDS activism's most misunderstood man (2). **INSIDE:** Canada's Supreme Court upholds the criminalization of people living with HIV for nondisclosure before consensual sex; a look at Steve Hart's deeply emotional photo essay *A Bronx Family Album: The Impact of AIDS.* **PLUS:** Larry Kramer and David Webster write about how they found love in an epidemic.

March

COVER: Olympic gold medalist Greg Louganis dives into dog training and shares an excerpt from his new book, *For the Life of Your Dog.* **INSIDE:** Actress Kathy Najimy on why she supports organizations such as LA Shanti and Project Angel Food. **PLUS:** The impact of provocative writer and artist David Wojnarowicz (3).

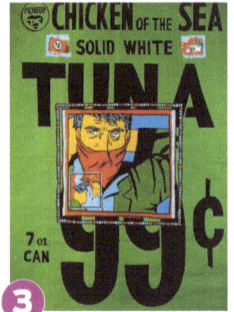

April

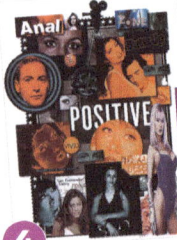

COVER: After Tricia Devereaux and four other adult film stars tested HIV positive, the straight porn industry is forced to react (4). **INSIDE:** The high cost of the latest HIV meds may bankrupt drug assistance programs; finding relief from wasting and lipodystrophy. **PLUS:** How to make art in an epidemic.

May

COVER: For POZ's fifth anniversary, we catch up with past cover subjects Moisés Agosto, Rebekka Armstrong, Shawn Decker, Kiyoshi Kuromiya, Raven Lopez, Ty Ross, Andrew Sullivan and Susan Rodriguez. **INSIDE:** Authors, artists and activists reflect on the current state of HIV; the long-term side effects of protease inhibitors (5). **PLUS:** The HAART Chart breaks down the incidence rates of med side effects.

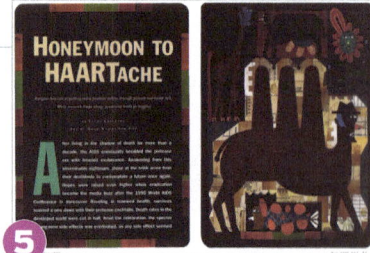

June

COVER: A report on how advances in prevention science could revolutionize safer sex. **INSIDE:** Tips for talking to doctors or nurses about your pain (6); POZ's Nurse Know-It-All offers advice for sun and sleep seekers. **PLUS:** Choreographer Muna Tseng's last dance with her older brother, photographer Tseng Kwong Chi.

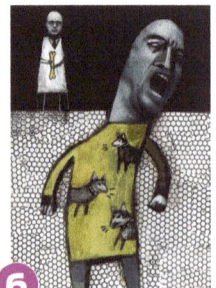

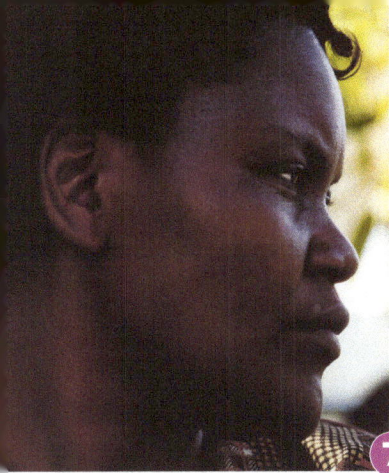

July

COVER: Guest-edited by Phill Wilson, our special "In Africa" issue highlights the crisis on the continent. **INSIDE:** Advocating for the expansion of scientific research into how gender differences affect antiretroviral dosing, resistance, side effects and more. **PLUS:** Scovia Kazolo is a Ugandan nurse-midwife living with HIV who melds modern medicine with traditional healing (**7**).

August

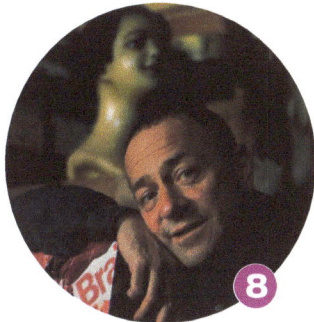

COVER: A look inside the curious closets of artist Barton Lidice Beneš—you never know what or whom you'll find (**8**). **INSIDE:** Puerto Rican officials are accused of embezzling federal AIDS funds; how to prevent parasites—and treat them. **PLUS:** Special summer fiction: Richard McCann's short story on love and loss.

September

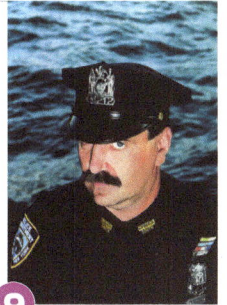

COVER: NYPD officer Steve Yurcik was surprised by the support he received from his fellow officers in blue when he disclosed his HIV status (**9**). **INSIDE:** Immigrants living with HIV who are detained by the Immigration and Naturalization Service may face unpredictable health care. **PLUS:** An interview with *Where the Wild Things Are* author Maurice Sendak, whose cherished drawings have been turned into a wall-sized mural at GMHC in New York City.

October

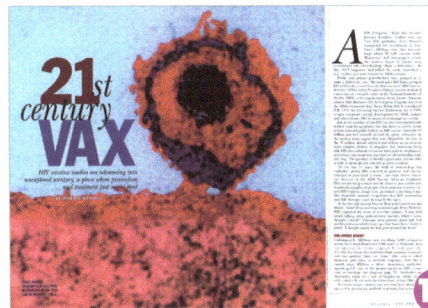

COVER: Researcher Steven Miles on why the protease boom went bust—and what we can do about it. **INSIDE:** The search for a vaccine advances into uncharted territory and may be found where prevention and treatment intersect (**10**); transgender activists are fighting to make the system work for their sisters and brothers. **PLUS:** Tibor Kalman's graphic activism in Colors magazine.

November

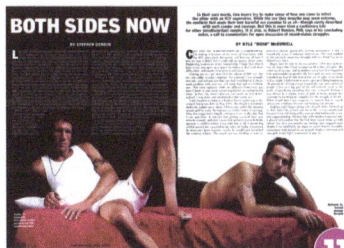

COVER: In their own words, Stephen Gendin and Hush McDowell try to make sense of how one came to transmit an HIV supervirus to the other (**11**). **INSIDE:** A community action agenda on how to end the epidemic; if you're tired and cranky and lost your love mojo, you might blame it on your hormones. **PLUS:** Transgender nun Sister Mary Elizabeth is the wizard behind AEGIS— the AIDS Education Global Information System, the largest HIV website in the world.

December

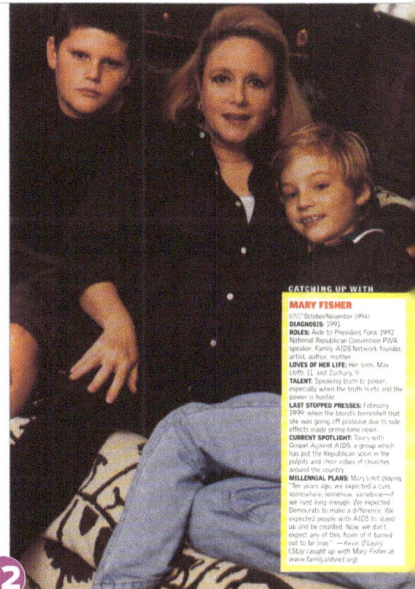

COVER: From riots to ribbons, 99 monumental moments of the AIDS epidemic during the '90s. **INSIDE:** A guide to the new world of adherence high anxiety; catching up with former cover subject Mary Fisher (**12**); will a structured treatment interruption make your holiday season jolly, or is it a folly? **PLUS:** Meet Ferd Eggan, Los Angeles's radical AIDS czar.

Antiretrovirals:
A Success Story

CELEBRATING 20 YEARS OF EFFECTIVE HIV TREATMENT

BY
BENJAMIN RYAN

N EARLY 1996, JEFFREY Pope began getting his affairs in order, straightening out his finances and his home and visiting his parents for what he assumed would be the last time.

"I was preparing to die," Pope says. Since his AIDS diagnosis the previous year, he'd seen his CD4 count plunge from a healthy 600 to a precarious

170. He weathered shingles, pneumocystis pneumonia (PCP) and bouts of severe flu. He had to stop working. The antiretrovirals (ARVs) he was taking— either one or two nucleoside reverse transcriptase inhibitors (NRTIs, or nukes) at a time, ... was standard during the early 1990...

By April ... out, ar ... keep ...

A ... trip ... ne ...

the first drug from a ne... protease inhibitors (PI)... joined the legion of p... who benefited from... Lazarus syndrome— at life.

In July 1996, ir... perts from aroun... in Vancouver for... AIDS Confere... these gatherin... ...g, as data ... ...the

---

Victory

FDA warns that prote...

BY

n June, the Food and ... Administration (FDA) issu... nationwide warning that ... tease inhibitors may cause ... vated blood sugar (hy... glycemia) and even diabetes in p... ple with HIV. Still, many questi... remain about how the drugs are c... nected to the effect, and how sever... risk they pose.

The warning was issued after t... agency received 83 reports of new ... exacerbated diabetes mellitus ... increased blood-sugar levels in patien... taking protease inhibitors. Six cas... were life-threatening and 21 require... hospitalization. Many of the case... reversed when patients stopped takin... the drugs—but not all. The high bloo... sugar was often controlled with addi... tional oral drugs or insulin injections

All four of the currently approved ... protease inhibitors were implicated. ... "It looks like the number of cases ... [for each drug] was roughly paral- ... lel to prescription usage," FDA ... medical officer Jeff Murray says. ... The FDA has estimated high ... blood sugar may occur in as ... few as 0.1 percent to 1 ... percent of people ... using protease in- ... hibitors—rare ... enough that ... the problem ... was not recog- ... nized in clini- ... cal drug trials. ... Nonetheless, ... the FDA ordered ... manufacturers of ... all four drugs to ... change product labels to warn about ... the potential side effect.

Not all those who develop diabetes ... have pre-existing risk factors. Robin ... Dretler, MD, senior partner at ... Infectious Disease Specialists in ... Atlanta, has treated one case of dia- ... betes in a man takin...

POZ
HEALTH, LIFE & HIV

HIV DRUG CHART

Antiretroviral (ARV) options abound for bot... are new to HIV treatment and tho... This quick-reference chart com... options, including dosing and d...

Single Tablet Regimens

ATRIPLA
(efavirenz + tenofovir + emtricitabine)
One tablet once a day. Contains two NRTIs and one NNRTI in one tablet.
Take on an empty stomach and at bedtime to minimize dizziness, drowsiness and impaired concentration.

COMPLERA
(rilpivirine + tenofovir + emtricitabine)
One tablet once a day. Contains two NRTIs and one NNRTI in one tablet.
Take with a meal containing fat.

STRIBILD
(elvitegravir + cobicistat + tenofovir + emtricitabine)
One tablet once a day. Contains two NRTIs, one integrase inhibitor and one pharmacokinetic (PK) enhancer in one tablet.
Take with food.

Reverse Transcriptase Inhibitors (NRTIs)

INTELENCE
(etravirine)
One 200 mg tablet twice a day, or two 100 mg tablets twice a day.
Take with food.

EDURANT
(rilpivirine)
One 25 mg tablet once a day.
Take with a meal containing fat.

SUSTIVA
(efavirenz)
One 600 mg tablet once a day, or three 200 mg capsules once a day.
Take on an empty stomach and at bedtime to minimize dizziness, drowsiness and impaired concentration.

VIRAMUNE XR
(nevirapine)
One 200 mg Viramune IR tablet once a day for the first 14 days, then one 400 mg Viramune XR tablet once a day.

Integrase Inhibitors

ISENTRESS
(raltegravir)
One 400 mg tablet twice a day.
Take with or without food.

TIVICAY
(dolutegravir)
One 50 mg tablet once a day for those starting ARV therapy for the first time or for those who have not used an integrase inhibitor in the past. One 50 mg tablet twice a day for those who are resistant to the first-generation integrase inhibitors and when taken with certain ARVs.
Take with or without food.

Fusion and Entry Inhibitors

FUZEON
(enfuvirtide)
One 90 mg injecti...
Fuzeon comes as a ... that must be mixed ... water in a vial each d... being injected.
Take with or without fo...

SELZENTRY
(maraviroc)
One 150 mg tablet, one 300 mg tablet, or two 300 mg tablets twice a day (because Selzentry interacts ... HIV drugs, the dose will
*not...

25 Years of HIV Research

THE INCREASING MASTERY OVER THE VIRUS IS ONE OF HUMANITY'S CROWNING ACHIEVEMENTS.

BY BENJAMIN RYAN

When POZ magazine was founded in 1994, the U.S. AIDS crisis was just reaching its peak. By the following year, half a million Americans had been diagnosed with the disease and nearly two thirds of them were already dead. And so, marrying the take-no-prisoners activism of ACT UP with the tenacious truth-seeking of a countercultural publication, POZ's scrappy staff and cadre of writers armed themselves with the power of the pen against a potentially indefinite holocaust.

Clockwise from top, coverage from POZ: feature story from the July/August 2016 issue, article from the October 1997 issue, drug chart from the July/August 2014 issue

Then came a miracle. In 1996, the first effective combination regimens to treat HIV became available, kick-starting the Lazarus era of the epidemic practically overnight. This reprieve was 15 years in the making—AIDS was first officially identified in 1981—and was the result of the dogged efforts of activists and scientists who were determined to outsmart one of the most destructive and wily viruses to affect the human race.

For a quarter-century now, POZ has provided readers a front-row seat to an astonishing parade of scientific advancements—as well as humbling setbacks—in the worldwide effort to control the global HIV pandemic. It's no hyperbole to claim that the ever-refined collective mastery that scientists have gained over the virus during this period represents one of the all-time greatest achievements of human ingenuity.

But the great work is only beginning. Quality of life for people living with HIV has certainly improved, but the challenges the thousands of HIV researchers toiling around the globe still face are mammoth and sprawling. Vanquishing this particular virus is not merely a matter of developing effective treatments, preventives, vaccines and cure therapies. Epidemic-ending success will require solving the byzantine sociocultural and geopolitical puzzles of how a microscopic sphere encasing a collection of RNA could exploit the myriad weaknesses and faults of societies in order to infect some 77 million people to date, killing nearly half of them.

If the past 25 years of scientific advancements in this field are any guide, the future looks bright.

Drug Development

Today, the bedrock of the fight against HIV is the healthy crop of 28 approved antiretrovirals (ARVs) that fall into five classes as well as the 13 single-tablet regimens (STRs) that require only once-daily dosing. For those with multidrug-resistant virus, the antibody therapy Trogarzo (ibalizumab) recently became available. Additionally, HIV regimens may include either of two "boosters," Norvir (ritonavir) and Tybost (cobicistat), which increase the levels of ARVs in the body.

During the contrastingly impoverished early 1990s, hopes that the paucity of ARVs available at the time would significantly extend the lives of people with AIDS were progressively dashed. It turned out that treating HIV with only one or two medications from the nucleoside/nucleotide reverse transcriptase inhibitor (NRTI) class—the first, Retrovir (zidovudine, or AZT), was approved in 1987—wasn't enough to beat back the virus. In fact, such treatment often wound up spawning

viral resistance to the medications, thus narrowing an individual's future treatment options.

Then, in December 1995, the Food and Drug Administration (FDA) approved Invirase (saquinavir), the first protease inhibitor. In June of the following year, Viramune (nevirapine) hit the market as the first non-nucleoside reverse transcriptase inhibitor (NNRTI). Finally, HIV clinicians could prescribe "cocktails" of three ARVs, which proved to be enough of a multipronged assault to render the virus undetectable in the body—as confirmed by the newly approved viral load test.

Between 1996 and 1997, AIDS deaths plummeted 47% in the United States.

The rub was that some of those ARVs were highly toxic and caused devastating side effects, such as lipodystrophy and diabetes. Additionally, treating HIV required taking numerous pills per day according to rigid schedules and onerous food-intake protocols. Such burdens compromised people's adherence to their ARV regimens, which in turn fueled viral rebound and resistance.

The 2000s brought increasing relief as newer drugs proved ever more tolerable and simpler to take and required less strict adherence to keep viral resistance at bay. Atripla (efavirenz/tenofovir disoproxil fumarate/emtricitabine) was

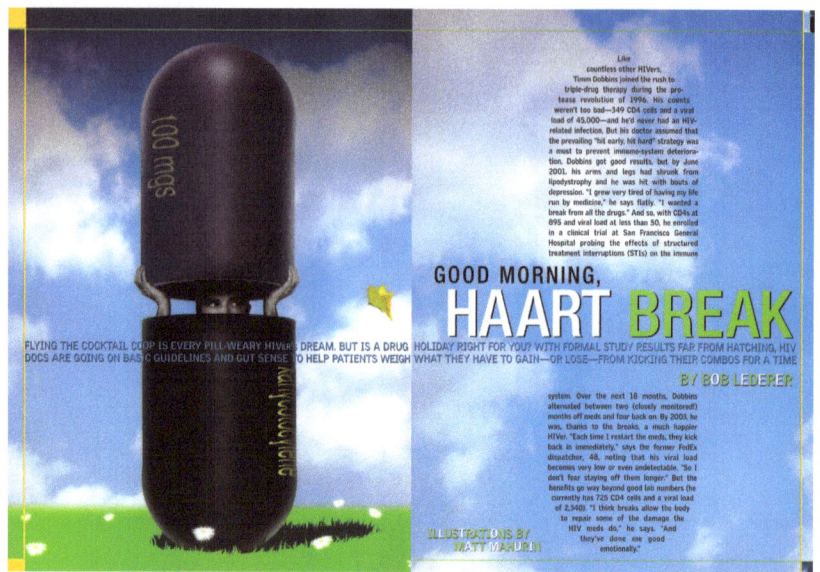

GOOD MORNING, HAART BREAK
BY BOB LEDERER

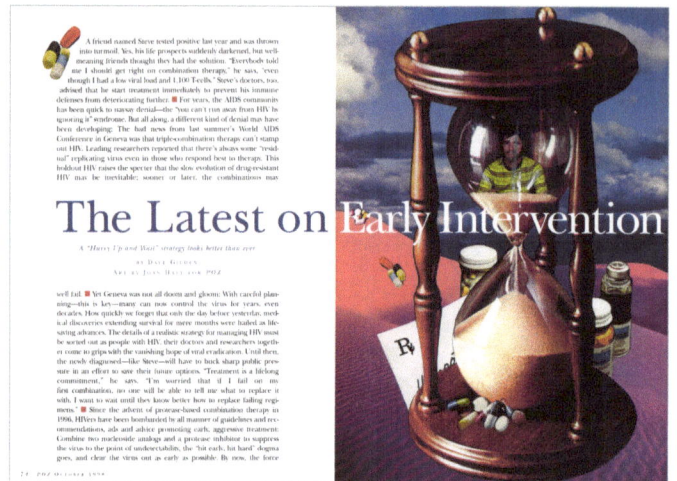

The Latest on Early Intervention

Top: coverage from the April 2003 issue; bottom: from the October 1998 issue

PREVIOUS PAGES: (FOLDER) ISTOCK

CAN PERSONAL CHOICE
AND PUBLIC HEALTH
FIND COMMON GROUND
IN PRE-EXPOSURE
PROPHYLAXIS?

PrEP AND PREJUDICE

BY BENJAMIN RYAN

A GROWING GLOBAL COMMUNITY
BUILDS A MOVEMENT.
BY OLIVIA G. FORD

Understanding Undetectable

Equals Untransmittable

approved in 2006 as the first STR. The following year, the FDA green-lit Isentress (raltegravir), the first of the well-tolerated and highly potent integrase inhibitors.

Thanks to these pharmaceutical advancements and improvements in the overall care of people with HIV, life expectancy for those on ARV treatment today is approaching normal. Nevertheless, researchers continue to refine and improve the HIV treatment tool kit.

The past two years have seen the first STRs that include only two ARVs: Juluca (dolutegravir/rilpivirine) and Dovato (dolutegravir/lamivudine). A long-acting injectable regimen, dosed monthly, will likely gain approval in late 2019. And further down the road, long-acting antibody treatments might require dosing as seldom as two to four times per year.

Top: pre-exposure prophylaxis coverage from the October/November 2014 issue; bottom: Undetectable Equals Untransmittable coverage from the March 2019 issue

The Treatment-Initiation Conundrum

At the dawn of the triple-combination ARV era, "hit early, hit hard" was the defining treatment ethos—influenced, in part, by a faulty belief that long-term fully suppressive therapy would eventually cure HIV. In 1998, the Department of Health and Human Services (HHS) recommended starting ARVs once an individual's CD4 count had dropped to 500 or below.

Three years later, in an effort to spare people with HIV the devastating side effects of those early ARVs as much as possible and also to mitigate the emergence of drug resistance, HHS did an about-face. The agency now advised ARV treatment only after CD4s had dropped to an AIDS-defining 200 or lower.

During these trying times, various studies found that people could take periodic breaks, known as drug holidays, from their ARV regimens without lasting immune-system damage. The randomized controlled SMART study, launched in 2002, aimed to confirm such findings using gold-standard research. But in 2006, the landmark trial was terminated years ahead of schedule because it had become evident that drug holidays were actually associated with a higher risk of HIV disease progression and death.

SMART's stunning findings rocked the HIV research world, in particular because of the discovery that interrupting treatment fueled harmful inflammation—which is itself associated with various health risks. The study ultimately set the stage for the randomized controlled START trial, which began in 2011 and sought to determine whether there was a net health benefit to beginning ARVs with CD4s above 500 versus waiting until the count declined to 350 or below.

In an episode of randomized-controlled-trial déjà vu, the START administrators canceled that study's deferred-treatment arm in 2015, more than a year ahead of schedule. Going on HIV treatment early, it had already become clear, reduced the risk of AIDS-defining illnesses and other serious maladies. (The trial continues to monitor participants to assess any differences in long-term health outcomes between those who started treatment immediately and those who did so on a delayed basis.)

Upon the START trial's release, HHS, which had raised the CD4 threshold for an ARV initiation recommendation to 350 CD4s in 2008 and then to 500 CD4s in 2010, promptly advised universal treatment regardless of CD4 count.

After two decades, the HIV treatment protocol had come full circle.

Prevention

Most of the HIV prevention modalities developed since the early years of the epidemic, when condoms were the only option, are based upon what's known as the biomedical prevention of HIV—the use of medications to thwart transmission.

A major study released in 1994 found that giving AZT to pregnant women with HIV prevented mother-to-child transmission of the virus. Not long after that drug's 1987 release, health care workers began taking a course of ARVs following a potential exposure to HIV on the job.

By 2005, enough research supported the use of post-exposure prophylaxis (PEP)—in which an individual starts a month of a triple-ARV regimen within 48 to 72 hours of a potential exposure to HIV—for the Centers for Disease Control and Prevention (CDC) to finally expand its PEP guidelines to include sexual as well as occupational exposure.

Research findings from the mid-1990s indicated that syringe services programs providing clean needles and syringes to people who inject drugs reduced their risk of HIV.

Beginning in 2011, a trio of major studies, HPTN 052, PARTNER and Opposites Attract, released a progressive avalanche of data supporting the hypothesis that successful HIV treatment prevents transmission. By the time PARTNER announced findings from its second phase in 2018, a global scientific consensus had solidified: People with HIV who maintain an undetectable viral load cannot transmit the virus through sex.

Meanwhile, in 2010, the randomized controlled iPrEx study found that people not living with HIV who took Truvada (tenofovir disoproxil fumarate/emtricitabine) as pre-exposure prophylaxis (PrEP) greatly reduced their risk of getting HIV. Researchers would subsequently estimate that daily use of the tablet cuts the risk of HIV by more than 99% among men who have sex with men (MSM) and by at least 90% among women. More recently, the French IPERGAY study confirmed that taking Truvada doses only during the 72-hour period surrounding the time of sex is also highly effective as PrEP for MSM.

By the end of 2019, the FDA will likely approve a new PrEP option: Descovy (tenofovir alafenamide/emtricitabine), which has the same components as Truvada but with an updated version of the drug tenofovir that is linked to improved markers of bone and kidney health. (It is not known whether using Descovy over Truvada would actually prevent fractures or kidney disease.) A long-acting injectable form of PrEP given every eight weeks may also hit the market by about 2023. Researchers are further investigating long-acting antibody shots as PrEP and, much further back in the pipeline, implants that slowly release preventive medication over a period of months.

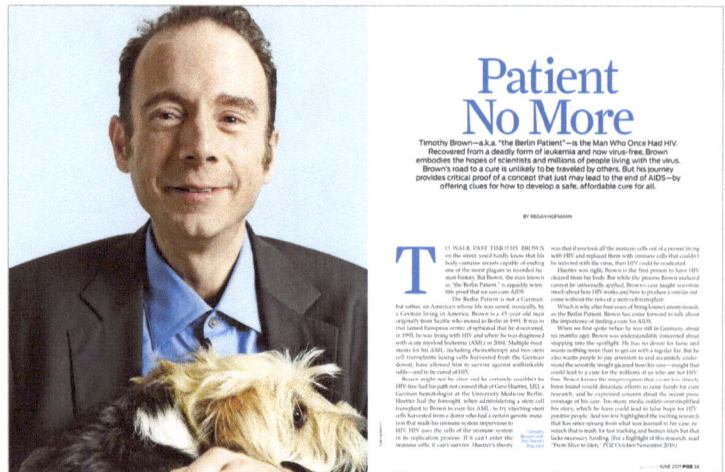

Top: coverage of "the Berlin Patient" from the June 2011 issue; bottom: update on cure research from the January/February 2019 issue

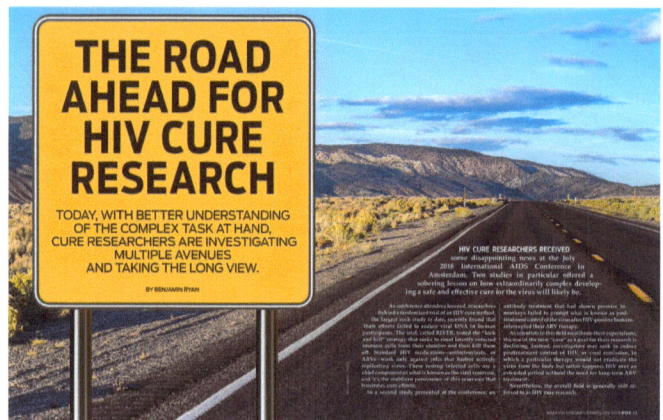

The quest for an HIV vaccine has proved particularly frustrating, beset as it has been with repeated failures of major research efforts since the first Phase III trial launched in 1998. Only a single late-stage vaccine study—conducted in Thailand and published in 2009—showed any efficacy: a 31% reduction in HIV risk. Investigators have since sought to build on that result and develop a more potent product. Today, two late-stage trials of vaccines are under way, and experts are hopeful the candidates will prove at least 50% effective—powerful enough to justify a global rollout by the mid-2020s.

A trio of randomized controlled trials conducted in sub-Saharan Africa and published in the mid-aughts found that voluntary medical male circumcision lowered the risk of female-to-male HIV transmission by about 60%. This finding has led to a concerted push to circumcise millions of males throughout the continent, which has been tied to declining HIV rates among both women and men.

After decades of efforts to develop microbicides to prevent HIV—ARV-infused gels, inserts, rectal douches and the like—researchers have suffered numerous stumbles and setbacks and have succeeded in developing only one such product thus far: a monthly vaginal ring. Currently awaiting regulatory approval, the ring provides at least a

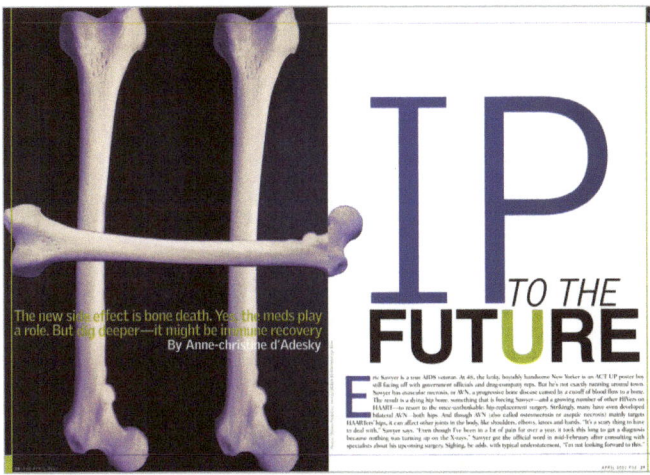

HIP TO THE FUTURE

The new side effect is bone death. Yes, the meds play a role. But dig deeper—it might be immune recovery

By Anne-christine d'Adesky

Top: from the April 2002 issue; bottom: from the June 2002 issue

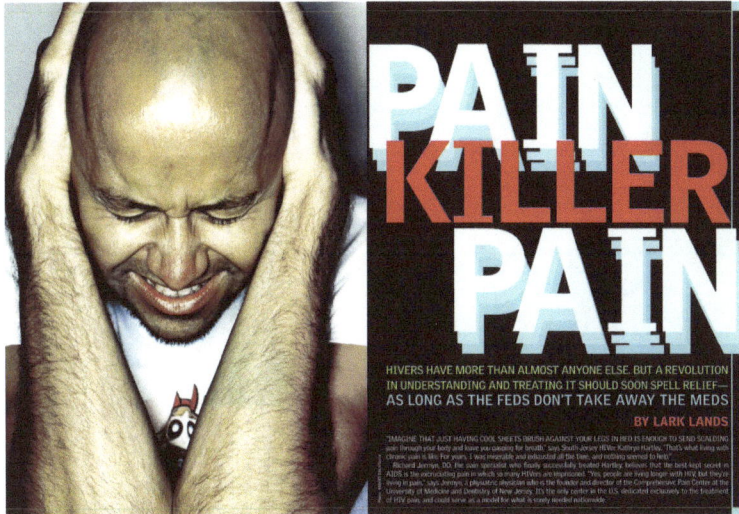

PAIN KILLER PAIN

HIVERS HAVE MORE THAN ALMOST ANYONE ELSE. BUT A REVOLUTION IN UNDERSTANDING AND TREATING IT SHOULD SOON SPELL RELIEF—AS LONG AS THE FEDS DON'T TAKE AWAY THE MEDS

BY LARK LANDS

modifying an individual's own cells in an attempt to foster an HIV-resistant immune system like Brown's—but without the need for potentially fatal cancer treatment such as he received. A third tactic is called "block and lock," the goal of which is to keep latently infected cells in an indefinite resting state so they never wake up and churn out new virus.

Other Health Conditions

Even when people with HIV maintain an undetectable viral load on ARVs, they have a higher risk of developing a host of conditions, many of which are related to aging but tend to strike those with the virus at ages younger than those seen among the general population. These health problems, the incidence of which is driven in part by the overall aging of the HIV population, include cardiovascular disease, various cancers, diabetes, high cholesterol and blood pressure, kidney and liver disease, chronic pain, cognitive decline, bone loss and gastrointestinal problems.

Scientists believe that the chronic inflammatory state associated with even well-treated HIV contributes to many of these outcomes. A major ongoing randomized controlled trial called REPRIEVE, set to complete in 2023, is seeking to determine whether prescribing a cholesterol-lowering statin to people with HIV will temper such inflammation and in so doing reduce the risk of cardiovascular disease and various other health conditions as well as the risk of death.

The HIV population has high rates of other risk factors that fuel major diseases, in particular smoking, as well as coinfection with hepatitis B and C viruses (HBV and HCV). Fortunately, newer hepatitis C treatments have made HCV infection readily curable, and HBV is not only treatable but also vaccine preventable.

Additionally, ARVs themselves, especially the oldest ones, have been tied to myriad health problems. Mental illness and substance abuse disorders may also compromise the health and well-being of HIV-positive individuals.

Compounding all these negative impacts, many people with the virus are low-income and struggle with their basic needs, such as accessing proper food and nutrition, housing, transportation, child care and health care.

In response to such complex concerns, research into improving the care and treatment of HIV increasingly takes a cross-disciplinary, holistic approach that seeks to address the totality of each individual's unique needs. The ultimate goal is to provide the most robust and comprehensive support for those living with the virus in the hope that they don't just live a long and healthy life but truly thrive throughout the years. ■

modest level of protection against the virus. Meanwhile, U.S. funding priorities are shifting away from microbicide research, a change that calls into question the future of other such preventive products in the pipeline.

Cure

In 2008, the news that a man dubbed "the Berlin Patient" and later identified as Timothy Ray Brown had been cured of the virus jolted the once-sleepy HIV cure research field into action. As treatment for his leukemia, Brown had received stem cell transplants from a donor born with a genetic abnormality that rendered his immune cells resistant to HIV.

Members of the burgeoning HIV cure research field, backed by swelling financial support, are tasked with the challenge of outsmarting a virus that hides in long-lived resting immune cells. Collectively known as the viral reservoir, these latently infected immune cells remain under the radar of standard ARV treatment, which works only on actively replicating cells.

The long road toward achieving some form of widely replicable cure, viral remission or post–ARV treatment control of HIV is currently following several paths. One strategy, called "kick and kill," seeks to roust latent cells from their slumber and then finesse the immune system into attacking such cells. Another approach involves genetically

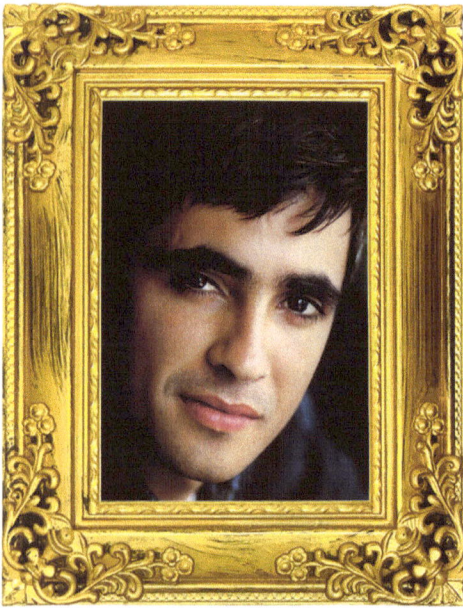

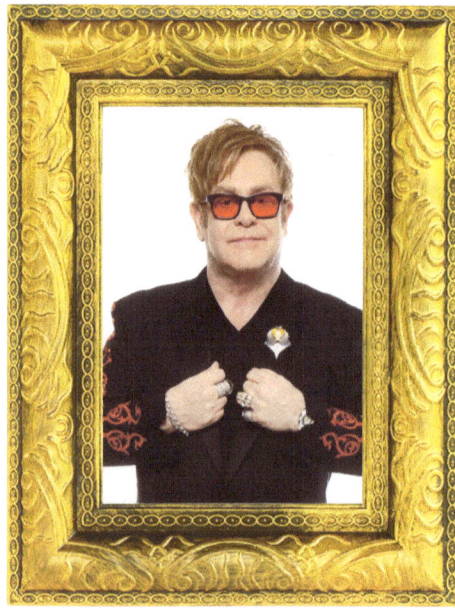

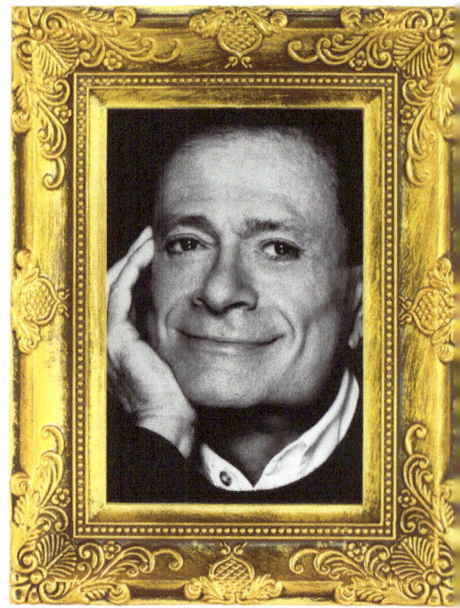

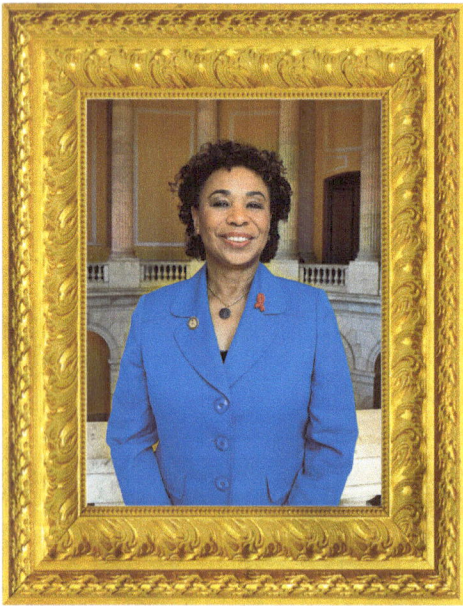

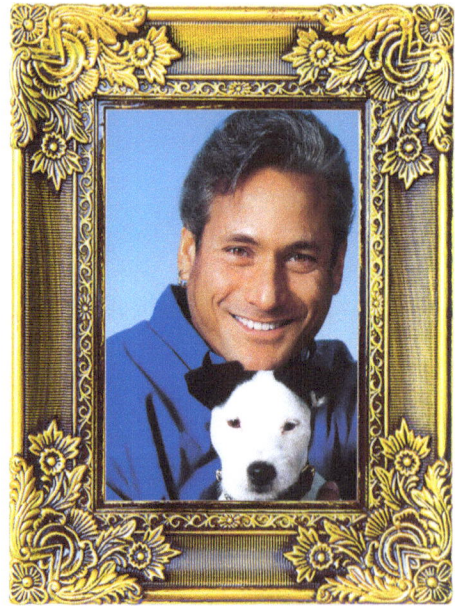

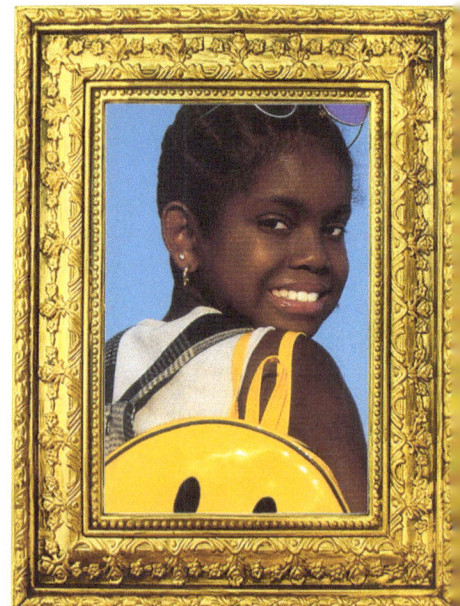

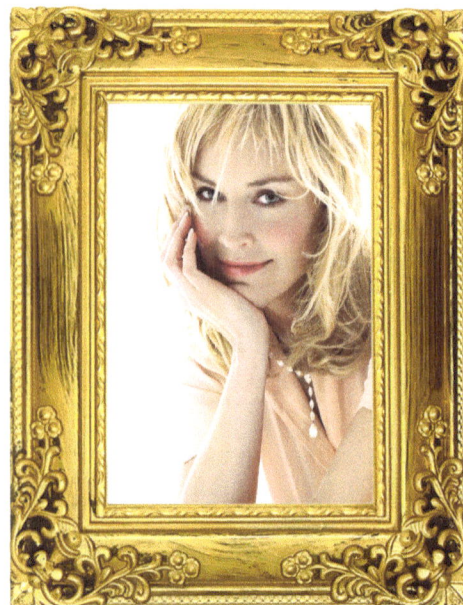

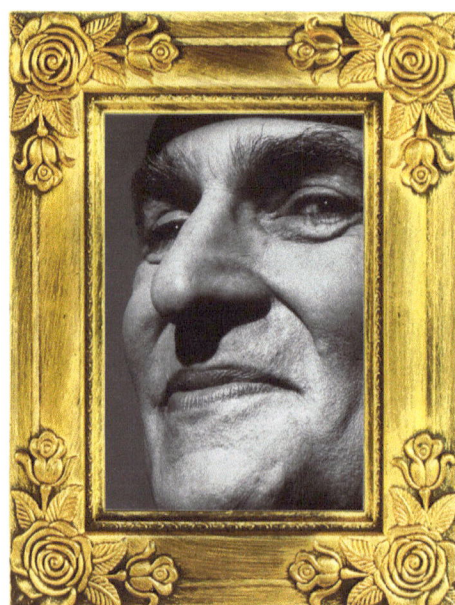

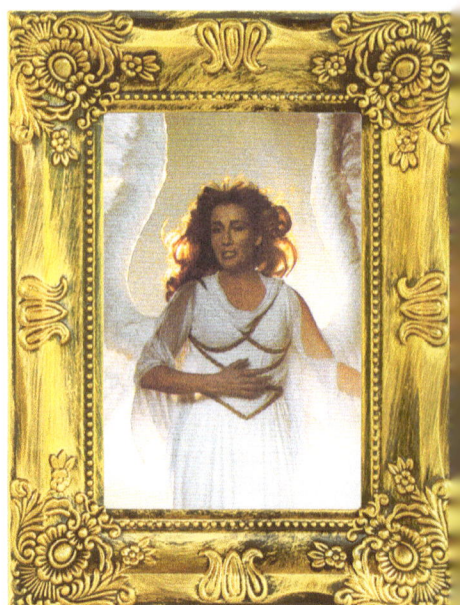

25 Years of Celebrities

OUR ESTEEM FOR THEIR HIV ACTIVISM—FROM THE RED CARPET TO BEYOND—IS A CONSTANT.

BY MARK S. KING

Celebrity is a curious thing. It is an exalted state of being that doesn't apply only to movie stars or the glamorous creatures on the red carpet. Celebrities are often beloved not because they have fame and fortune beyond our reach but because they might be us. In their faces we can see ourselves, wrapped in a different package, perhaps, but fighting hard for something we, too, believe in.

Coverage from POZ—left, top row: Pedro Zamora, Elton John, Jerry Herman; middle row: Barbara Lee, Greg Louganis, Hydeia Broadbent; bottom row: Sharon Stone, Larry Kramer, Emma Thompson; right: Elizabeth Taylor

FRAMES: ISTOCK

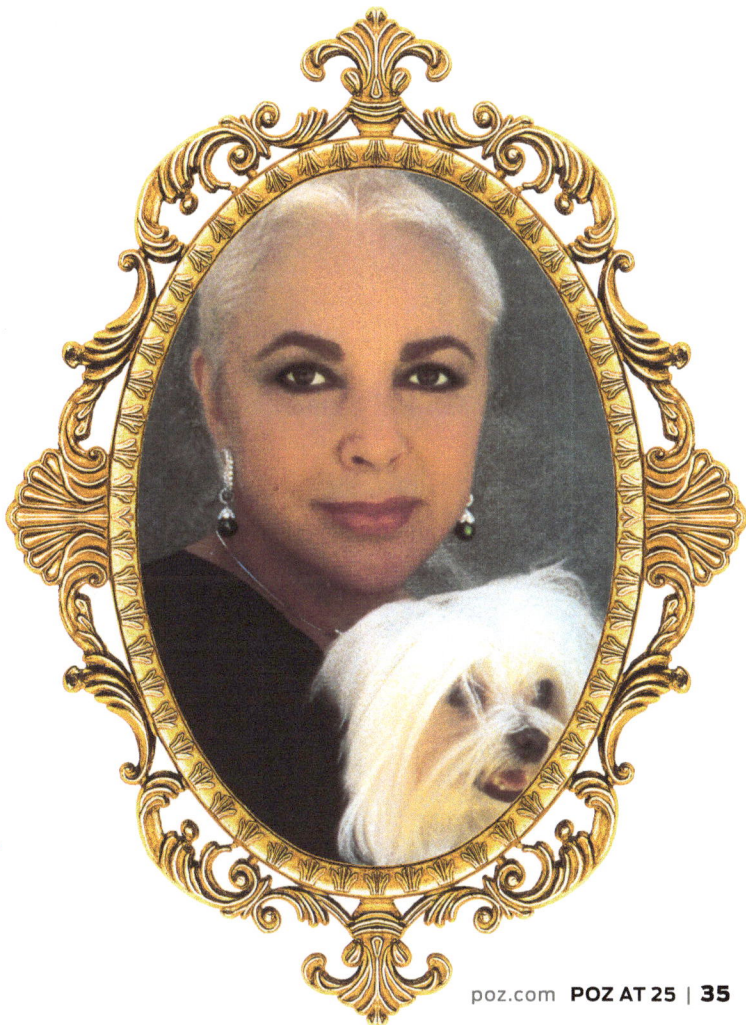

That is especially true in the HIV arena. We bestow celebrity status to community-based heroes as much as to the famous because we know the courage it takes to speak out as a person living with HIV or to stand up for us as an ally.

The people chosen to grace the covers of POZ through the years are a testament to these qualities. They might be a celebrity from Hollywood or sports, an AIDS activism icon or an emerging advocate bringing new energy to the field. Our esteem and gratitude for them is a constant.

Pedro Zamora appeared on the third issue of POZ and brought with him celebrity in all the forms we admire. He was a newly minted television star, appearing on MTV's hot new reality show, *The Real World*, and he was an HIV advocate finding his voice and using his new national platform. He disclosed his status as a gay man living with HIV to an enormous TV audience, and, over the course of a few episodes, he became a star.

Zamora was beautiful. He left us breathless. He knew who he wanted to be and the impact he wanted to have. Only months after he appeared on the August/September 1994 issue of POZ, Zamora died of AIDS-related complications at age 22. The world mourned along with us because he allowed us all to get to know him with all the intimacy the new genre of reality TV allowed. Everyone, it seemed, was a little bit in love with Zamora.

Larry Kramer, the godfather of ACT UP and GMHC, was photographed in stark black-and-white on the April/May 1995 cover, and he was grinning. It was a cheeky expression for a man so famous for his righteous anger, and the first of three cover appearances the mercurial writer and activist would make.

Conservative social critic Andrew Sullivan wrote the first Kramer cover story (Kramer would return the favor for Sullivan's cover story two years later), in which Sullivan has a meeting of the minds with Kramer, with whom he often disagrees. "Whatever history makes of Larry Kramer's role in this epidemic," Sullivan wrote, "it will have to record that...Larry Kramer was right."

The world of sports was delivered a shocking blow when basketball star Magic Johnson announced in 1991 that he was HIV positive and retiring. For advocates, the news was met with conflicting emotions: deep empathy for a man who was dealing with his new diagnosis and a sense of curiosity about how one of the most famous sports stars in the world might use this as an opportunity to educate and fight HIV stigma.

He eventually formed the Magic Johnson AIDS Foundation, but the normalcy of what he did in the years that followed his announcement changed public perceptions of people living with HIV. Johnson unretired, got back on the court and went on with his life.

"America remains largely ignorant about the nuances of the epidemic, but watching Magic Johnson play major-

Andrew Sullivan is, for many of us, a man of mystery. In his native Britain, he'd probably be just one of many eccentrics that country prides itself on harboring. Perhaps that's why he chooses to live in America. I like Andrew. I'm not certain, though, if I can tell you why. He has a nice smile. He's cute, sort of a gay Ralph Reed (though Ralph Reed always looks gay to me). And of course there's that British (or is it Oxford?) accent that's always so winning on this side of the Atlantic. My problem with Andrew is I have difficulty understanding what he stands for, what he believes in, what he wants us to think and do. I'm uncertain what his basic text is. His message, whatever it is, is unclear. Perhaps the best analogy I can think of is that when I hear or read Andrew—particularly when we're trying to define ourselves to each other—I feel like I'm talking to someone not speaking the same language I am. I don't mean a language like Urdu or Romanian. I mean a language like the biochemistry of newts. I tried to read his book, *Virtually Normal: An Argument for the Acceptance of Homosexuality.* I kept getting lost. I believe writing is about trying to make a case to the reader. I didn't understand Andrew's case. Even after reading a piece he wrote for *The New Republic* about why he didn't like me or ACT UP, I couldn't tell you what he didn't like about me or why he didn't approve of ACT UP. I just knew he didn't. And I was surprised when he told me that wasn't the case at all. Is this some sort of special gift he has, an ability to be imprecise with such precision that he'll soon become editor of *The New York Times*? Or is this a tragic flaw he has that keeps someone with such potential from becoming what we need more than anything: A gay, HIV positive spokesperson, fresh, smart, personable, with access to the media and those in positions of power? I worry that Andrew represents something very typical of this moment in history: An inability to precisely enunciate the issues, to precisely identify our enemies and to draw concrete suggestions of what we must do. But then perhaps I'm trying too hard to make him into what I try to do myself: Get out there on the line and give everyone hell for allowing the world to be such a shitty place for people with HIV. But

The world's most famous gay Catholic has deeply rooted convictions about God and country. His fears run pretty deep, too

BY LARRY KRAMER

PHOTOGRAPH BY ALBERT WATSON
EXCLUSIVELY FOR POZ

Rugged Andy: "I unveiled a great deal with my own conscience about the level to which I should be [out]."

"Openly HIV positive people are the recipients of all sorts of strange emotions."

Andrew Sullivan, True Believer

58 POZ April 1997   April 1997 POZ 59

Larry Kramer, With

Sugar

On Top

We all know Larry Kramer, or think we know him. The father of AIDS activism, the writer of the groundbreaking play, *The Normal Heart*, the founder of Gay Men's Health Crisis (GMHC) and then ACT UP, the pain in the ass of most AIDS organizations, the hysteric and sexy. I'd read his stuff before and found most of it unconvincingly shrill. But his early novel, *Faggots*, had struck a chord. It exuded a sense that gay men could do better if they understood themselves as fully human, if they could shed their self-loathing and self-deception. In Kramer's later work, I found—between the hyperbole and irresponsibility—a stark belief in the equality of lesbians and gay men and a conviction that AIDS was allowed to spread because of the people it first attacked. Both beliefs carried the unmistakable mark of truth. It was truth we all knew, but few of us had the clarity of mind or facility with words to state it so baldly. Whatever history makes of Larry Kramer's role in this epidemic, it will have to record that on these central facts, Larry Kramer was right. Like Randy Shilts, he was right.

BY ANDREW SULLIVAN

PHOTOGRAPHS BY ALBERT WATSON EXCLUSIVELY FOR POZ

"You've left all this till now?"

Health, Hope & HIV

POZ

Magic Realism

Survival of a Superstar

BY BRUCE SCHOENFELD

"I don't let AIDS dominate my life."

league basketball has given us a deeper understanding about the possibilities of life with AIDS," wrote Bruce Schoenfeld in his 1996 POZ cover story about the athlete. "No other person with HIV has driven home that point so clearly; Johnson does it every working day."

The theater community has suffered massive losses over the years, so the ebullient face of Broadway composer Jerry Herman on a 1997 cover of POZ was a joyful, soothing balm. The tunesmith behind *Hello, Dolly!* credited the advent of protease inhibitors, a new class of HIV medications at that time, for his renewed vigor, and he expressed pride over his part in bringing the drugs to approval by the Food and Drug Administration (FDA).

"My medical records were sent to the FDA along with many hundreds of others to help get the drug approved," Herman said. "I think that's the best thing I've done for this world."

Speaking of joy, the wide-eyed exuberance of cover subject Hydeia Broadbent, who was all of 4 feet tall and 13 years

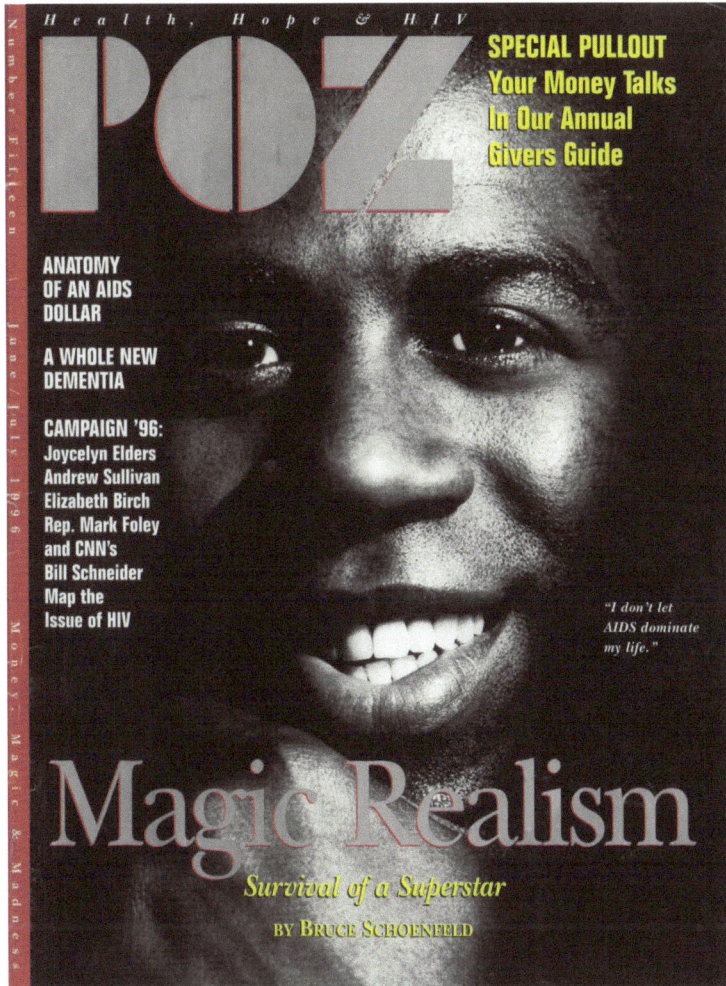

Left: Andrew Sullivan, Larry Kramer; above: Magic Johnson

old when she appeared on the October 1997 POZ cover, inspired readers everywhere. With a preternatural charm and intelligence, the barely-a-teen, who had been living with HIV since birth, made HIV education the mission of her young life.

Broadbent's cover story included her words in front of the 1996 Republican National Convention, spoken to a TV audience of millions. "I am the future, and I have AIDS," she said.

"I am Hydeia L. Broadbent. I can do anything I put my mind to. I am the next doctor. I am the next lawyer. I am the next Maya Angelou. I might even be the first woman president.... You can't crush my dream. I am the future, and I have AIDS."

The cover of POZ traditionally featured a person living with HIV on its cover—that is, until the November 1997 issue. That is the month that AIDS activist and film legend Elizabeth Taylor appeared on the cover in a photo taken by her close friend, actor Roddy McDowall.

All of Taylor's candor and beauty were on display in the cover story. Even while recuperating from brain surgery, Taylor remained feisty and laser-focused on her HIV advocacy. The founder of both The Elizabeth Taylor AIDS Foundation and amfAR, The American Foundation for AIDS Research, was reflective about the source of her altruism.

"I find being 'Elizabeth Taylor' really boring," she said. "I think if you were born with privileges—or given privileges—then you should share them. Like money—it's to share. I've known too many people who just sat and hoarded and were miserable. Just miserable SOBs. I have always believed that giving is one of the reasons that we were put on this earth."

The famously shy Olympian Greg Louganis opened up to POZ about his life more than 10 years after hitting his head on a diving board at the 1988 Olympics—and facing backlash when he revealed in his 1995 memoir that he was gay and living with HIV at the time of his accident.

By the time POZ featured Louganis on the cover in 1999, he had grown philosophical about the incident and the media frenzy that followed. "When the book came out, there were all these debates on blood in the pool and all that," Louganis said. "A lot of good information was getting out there, and that made me feel OK. It's important to know how you get HIV—and how you can't get it. And you cannot get HIV from a chlorinated pool."

Famed photographer Herb Ritts was known for his work behind the camera, but he took the spotlight on the cover of the April 2003 issue for a posthumous story about honesty in obituaries. Since the early days of AIDS, obituaries have often skirted the cause of death to protect the family or avoid HIV stigma. But Ritts's death from "pneumonia," as stated by his publicists, struck many as disingenuous.

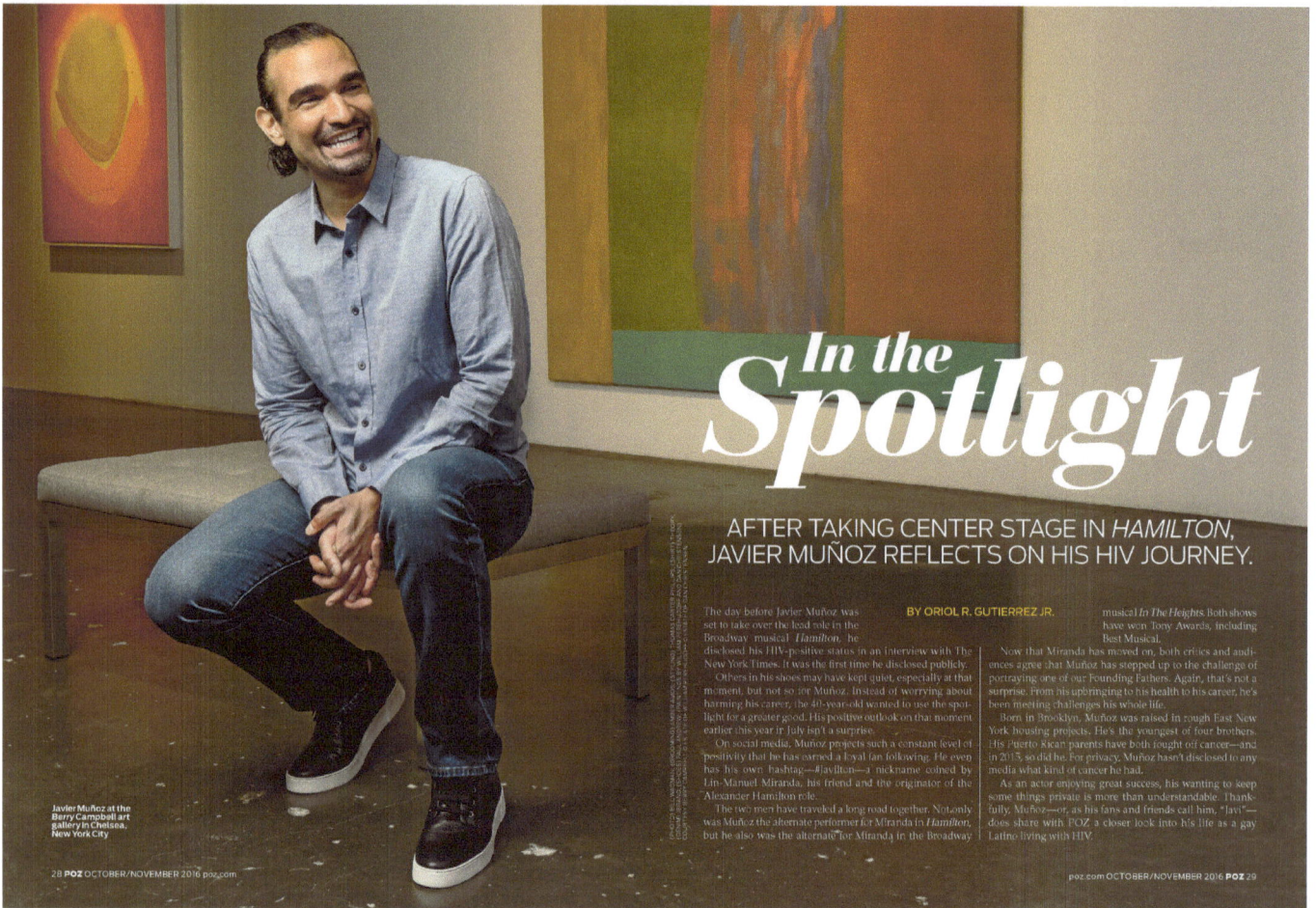

In the Spotlight

AFTER TAKING CENTER STAGE IN *HAMILTON*, JAVIER MUÑOZ REFLECTS ON HIS HIV JOURNEY.

BY ORIOL R. GUTIERREZ JR.

The day before Javier Muñoz was set to take over the lead role in the Broadway musical *Hamilton*, he disclosed his HIV-positive status in an interview with The New York Times. It was the first time he disclosed it publicly.

Others in his shoes may have kept quiet, especially at that moment, but not so for Muñoz. Instead of worrying about harming his career, the 40-year-old wanted to use the spotlight for a greater good. His positive outlook on that moment earlier this year in July isn't a surprise.

On social media, Muñoz projects such a constant level of positivity that he has earned a loyal fan following. He even has his own hashtag—#JavUton—a nickname coined by Lin-Manuel Miranda, his friend and the originator of the Alexander Hamilton role.

The two men have traveled a long road together. Not only was Muñoz the alternate performer for Miranda in *Hamilton*, but he also was the alternate for Miranda in the Broadway

musical *In The Heights*. Both shows have won Tony Awards, including Best Musical.

Now that Miranda has moved on, both critics and audiences agree that Muñoz has stepped up to the challenge of portraying one of our Founding Fathers. Again, that's not a surprise. From his upbringing to his health to his career, he's been meeting challenges his whole life.

Born in Brooklyn, Muñoz was raised in rough East New York housing projects. He's the youngest of four brothers. His Puerto Rican parents have both fought off cancer—and in 2015, so did he. For privacy, Muñoz hasn't disclosed to any media what kind of cancer he had.

As an actor enjoying great success, his wanting to keep some things private is more than understandable. Thankfully, Muñoz—or, as his fans and friends call him, "Javi"—does share with POZ a closer look into his life as a gay Latino living with HIV.

Javier Muñoz at the Berry Campbell art gallery in Chelsea, New York City

28 POZ OCTOBER/NOVEMBER 2016 poz.com

poz.com OCTOBER/NOVEMBER 2016 POZ 29

Top: Javier Muñoz; right: Elton John

LOVE IS THE CURE

WHEN IT COMES TO THE FIGHT AGAINST HIV, THE FOUNDER OF THE ELTON JOHN AIDS FOUNDATION BELIEVES WE NEED ALLIES, NOT ENEMIES.

34 POZ DECEMBER 2012

DECEMBER 2012 POZ 35

Nevertheless, outlets such as The New York Times repeated the claim without further questions.

"It was downright creepy to see a Reagan-era euphemism for AIDS pop up as the cause of Ritts's death in obituary after obituary," activist Michelangelo Signorile said in the piece. "Once again, this is a disease that dare not speak its name."

One of the most profound experiences in American theater of the late 20th century was arguably Tony Kushner's *Angels in America*, which took on mythic status for anyone who had the good fortune of seeing it onstage. An HBO production of the play, directed by Mike Nichols, became the lead subject of the December 2003 issue.

Emma Thompson appeared as the titular angel on the cover, representing an all-star cast that included Meryl Streep and Al Pacino. The trenchant drama, "a gay fantasia on national themes," blended big political debate with the intimacy of illness and death during the early AIDS crisis.

Actress Sharon Stone brought pure Hollywood glamour back to the cover in December 2007, in a story about her prodigious skills as a fundraiser for amfAR. Rather than push the tragic aspects of the epidemic, Stone was proving quite effective at using her high-wattage star power to encourage, charm and cajole major donors out of many millions of dollars.

38 | POZ AT 25 poz.com

Washington Warrior

Congresswoman Barbara Lee fearlessly leads the charge on Capitol Hill for people with HIV. Tens of millions of lives—including ours—depend on her ability to convince lawmakers to support the fight against AIDS. Having made an effective case for presidential leadership on the issue of ending AIDS, she now needs all the support she can get to rally the rest of Congress to champion the cause.

BY REGAN HOFMANN

Left: Herb Ritts; above: Barbara Lee

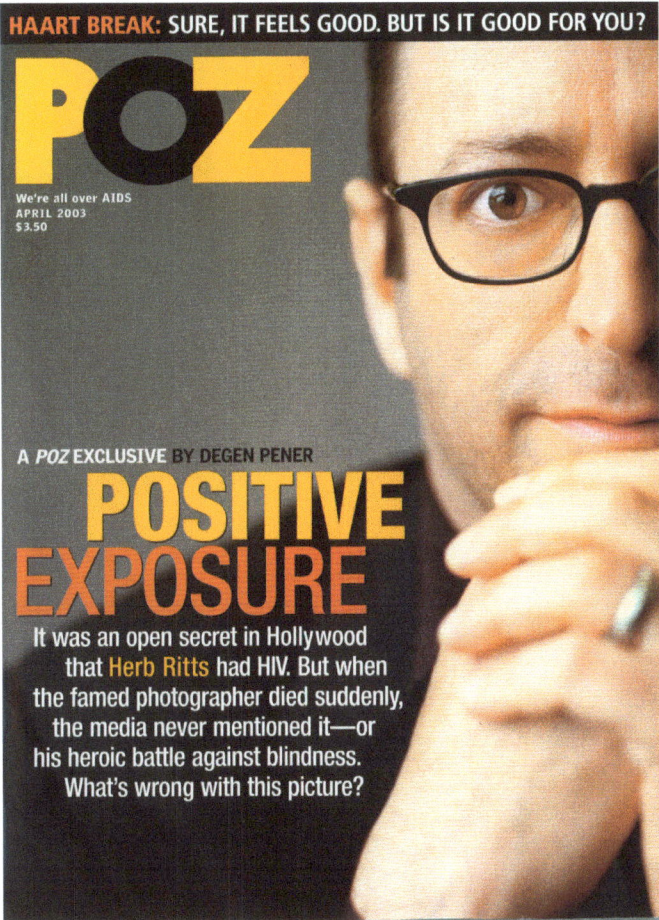

"She wields her beauty, her figure and her Hollywood persona to maximum effect," wrote editor-in-chief Regan Hofmann about the formidable star. "The mix is made all the more powerful by an ingredient especially compelling in a big blonde: big brains."

The power of Washington, DC, is an intoxicant as heady as all of Hollywood, and few things can be more effective than having a compelling political figure in your corner. The January/February 2012 cover story was a profile of Democratic Congresswoman Barbara Lee of California. The former social worker has made a political career of speaking up for the vulnerable and underserved.

Representative Lee was covered because of her agenda to get global aid to countries dealing with AIDS, make medications affordable in the United States and fight the unjust criminalization of people living with HIV. "Make no mistake," Lee said. "The world definitely has the money to end AIDS."

There are titans of the music industry, and then there are living legends like Elton John. A longtime friend and ally of people living with HIV, John appeared on the December 2012 issue on the occasion of the release of his book, *Love Is the Cure*. The memoir revisits his drug and alcohol addiction and recovery and how his friendship with teenager Ryan White inspired him to more fully commit to the fight against HIV.

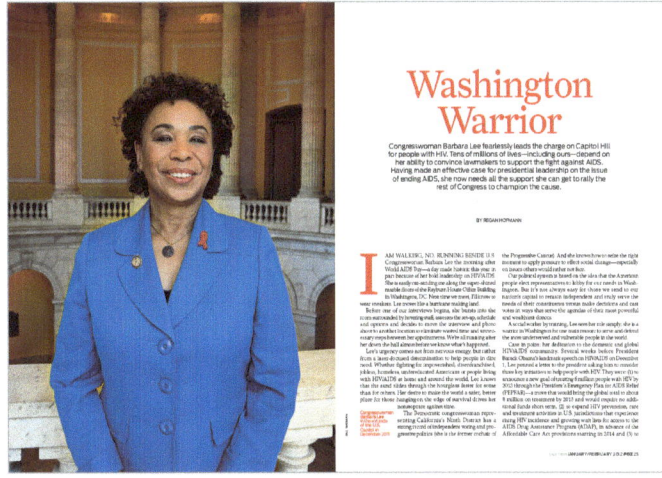

In the excerpt printed in POZ, John had the role of governments on his mind. "It is all too easy for political leaders to think about AIDS only in the abstract," he wrote. "It is all too easy for them to forget that there are real people counting on them for help, people who deserve the same chance to live a long life as anyone else."

The day before Broadway star Javier Muñoz took over the lead role in the musical phenomenon *Hamilton*, he told The New York Times he was living with HIV. There aren't many larger stages in the world on which to disclose your HIV status.

In his October/November 2016 cover story, Muñoz discussed his bold move. "I made the choice to disclose now to give hope to someone somewhere in this country or around the world who does not have the type of opportunities I've been given," he said. "There are still people who don't understand how the virus is transmitted. There are still people who don't understand what undetectable means. There's a bias that still exists. That to me is reason enough to be outspoken and to live out loud."

Standing alongside the big marquee names on the cover of POZ over the years are a legion of community advocates and newsmakers held in tremendous esteem by our community. To begin listing them would result in an avalanche of names, a veritable landslide of the deserving, the heroic, the game-changers and the grassroots advocates doing their work on the front lines every single day.

We know the people living with HIV speaking up at the planning meeting or the candlelight vigil. We watch them launch new programs, spread treatment news, tell their stories, lead a community. We see them on the pages of POZ, and we relate to them because we know what it means to stick our necks out, take a stand, risk rejection and speak up.

We look up to the stars, and we see ourselves. ◾

"Do you really want me naked?"

Ty Ross Comes Clea

BY KEVIN SESSUMS

Ty Ross, grandson of conservative icon Barry Goldwater, comes out for the first time as a HIV positive gay man and tackles homophobia, fame, politics and his own mortality.

Yet again: Los Angeles. I have visited here so often—either in my role as a journalist who specializes in celebrity interviews for *Vanity Fair* or as a guest of a few of my closest friends—that there is a comforting familiarity about the journey to my favorite hotel room at the Regent Beverly Wilshire from LAX, the very abbreviation of the city's airport confirming the laid-back attitude of the place. This trip is different, however. The person I am here to interview is not a celebrity in his own right, but the descendent of one. Ty Ross, the grandson of conservative icon Barry Goldwater, who ran for President the year that I turned 8 years old and the year that my mother died of cancer, has agreed to talk to me about being an HIV positive gay man. As the Hollywood hills come into view I think back to 1964 and how all three of us lost something that year—my mother, her life; Goldwater, his White House dream; I, my childhood. All journeys are personal ones, but this one, now 30 years later, will prove to be profoundly so.

Some Young Ty Ross in the early '80s when he first modeled for the Zoli agency in New York City.

PHOTOS GREG GORMAN FOR POZ. GROOMING: CHRIS MCMILLAN, PROFILES, LOS ANGELES, ASSISTANT: DAMIANO, PROFILES, LOS ANGELES

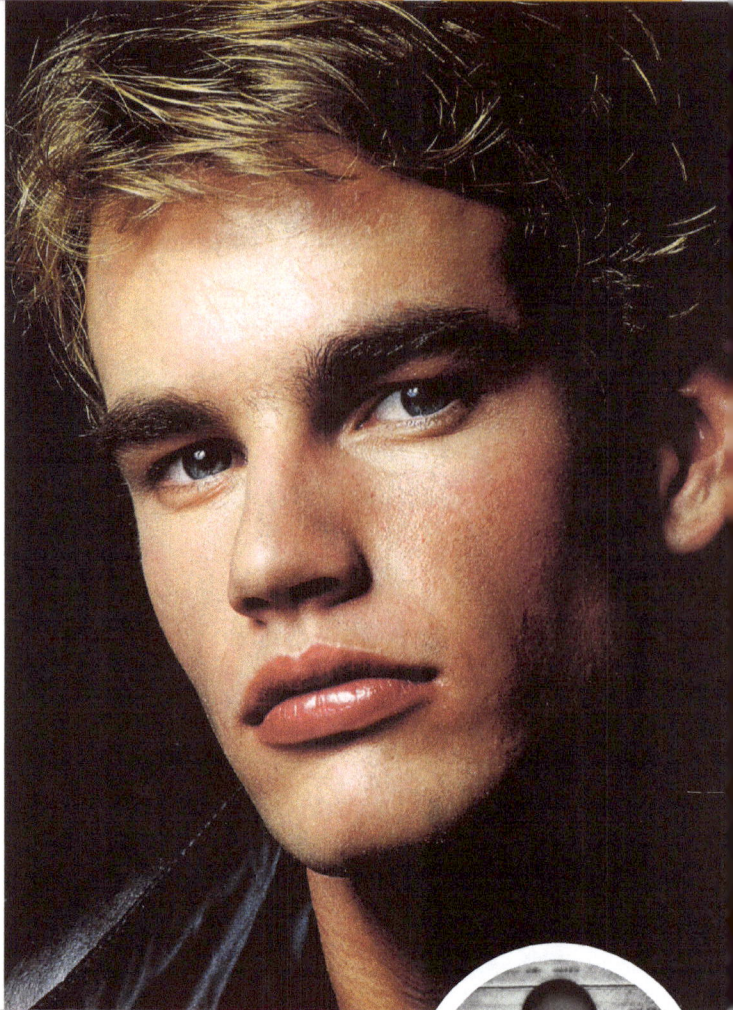

Hal Rubenstein
Interviewed Pedro Zamora

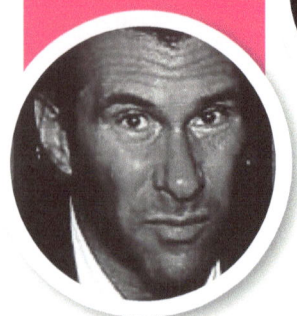

Chris Makos
Photographed Greg Louganis

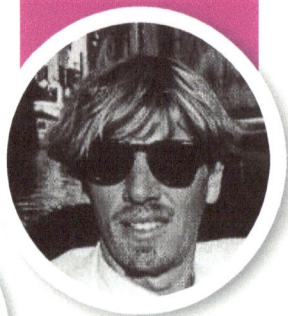

Maureen Dowd
Profiled Mary Fisher

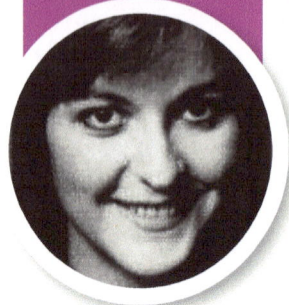

Mark Schoofs
Wrote a story about Jeffrey Schmalz

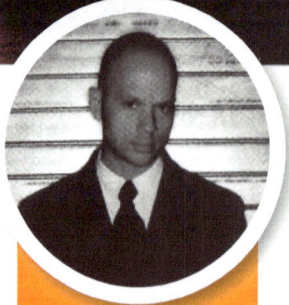

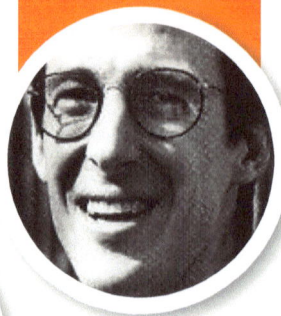

Kevin Sessums
Penned the cover story (above) for the first issue of POZ

25 Years of Contributors

POZ WRITERS AND ARTISTS HAVE THRIVED AT THE MAGICAL INTERSECTION OF LIVED EXPERIENCE AND BOUNDLESS TALENT.

BY TIM MURPHY

From that gorgeous, glossy debut issue in 1994, it must have been clear that when it came to contributing writers and artists, POZ would be no ordinary magazine.

The cover boy was Ty Ross, the photogenic HIV-positive grandson of conservative icon Barry Goldwater, and the writer was the equally adorable gay and HIV-negative Vanity Fair and Interview magazine hotshot Kevin Sessums.

The conclusion of their story was that subject and writer, having indulged in politically charged question-and-answer foreplay for hours, went to bed together. "We hold one another tightly before we begin to remove each other's clothes," wrote Sessums. "Naked, our bodies find the way that they must fit."

Well! Needless to say, the inaugural issue got more than a little attention. New York Times columnist Frank Rich called POZ "easily as plush as Vanity Fair" and "against all odds, the only new magazine of the year that leaves me looking forward to the next issue."

In those heady early years to come, the magazine boasted a roster of blue-chip contributors from all the best newspapers and magazines, including the Times, Vanity Fair, New York magazine, The Village Voice and then some. (Back then, the gay/downtown New York media universe was a small world. Everyone knew one another, and everyone wanted to be part of the fight against AIDS.)

New York Times superstar Maureen Dowd profiled HIV-positive Republican power player Mary Fisher. Mark Schoofs, who would go on to win a Pulitzer Prize for his Village Voice series on AIDS in Africa, wrote an appreciation of the pioneering openly gay and HIV-positive New York Times reporter Jeffrey Schmalz, who had just died of an AIDS-related illness. Style pundit Hal Rubenstein profiled MTV's *The Real World* heartthrob Pedro Zamora before Zamora was lost to AIDS in 1994. Warhol protégé Christopher Makos photographed HIV-positive Olympic diver Greg Louganis. The celebrity wattage was high.

But from day 1, POZ also balanced the boldface glitter with the real-life voices and wisdom of everyday folks living with HIV/AIDS, starting, of course, with its founder, Sean Strub, who in the first issue set out the magazine's manifesto by writing, "In my view, for a newly diagnosed person with AIDS, information is a more important first step than any pill, potion or prayer." And indeed, in every issue, at least half the content came directly from the pens (and, often, the lenses or drawing pencils) of HIV-positive folks themselves.

This roster included super wonky treatment know-it-alls like Gregg Gonsalves, Lark Lands, Mike Barr, Spencer Cox (died in 2012), Stephen Gendin (d. 2000), Mark Leydorf and Tim Horn, who wrote POZ's first feature on the coming protease inhibitor revolution.

But it also included a colorful stable of regular columnists writing on every aspect of daily life with the virus. "I have had the luxury of deciding whether to come out about my disease," wrote the fabulous Kiki Mason (d. 1996) about the divide between those who could and could not pass as healthy. "I haven't been forced out of the closet by wasting; my hair hasn't fallen out from chemo," he wrote. River Huston wrote about being a hetero female "sexpert" living with HIV, declaring, "I believe it is my karma to become a completely guilt-free, shame-free sexually expressive person."

"How can you have healthy people in a polluted environment?"

BY STEPHEN GRECO

Frank Moore

Call of the Wild

Frank Moore's art blends nature and medicine

"Débutantes," oil on canvas with attachments, 51 x 69" overall, 1992

Others included Dominic Hamilton-Little (d. 2011), David Feinberg (POZ's hilariously self-deprecating inaugural sex columnist until his death in 1994), and Shawn Decker, a young straight man from Virginia who contracted HIV from a blood product used to treat his hemophilia and went on to create an early blog, My Pet Virus, about daily life with HIV. "I've never smoked marijuana anyway, because I was always afraid it would lead to harsher drugs, like AZT," was a line typical of his adorably dorky sense of humor.

Over the years, more HIV-positive voices would join the POZ chorus. Joe Westmoreland and Bill Strubbe wrote comically yet honestly about the myriad health complications, side effects and emotional challenges of living with the virus. Shari Margolese wrote not only about being HIV-positive herself but also about raising an HIV-positive son. Mark Tuggle narrated his life as a gay Black man living with HIV, including getting sober and finding the doctor of his dreams. Beth Hastie wrote from the point of view of a lesbian living with HIV.

Brad Peebles, POZ's HIV-positive publisher in the late '90s and early 2000s, often wrote about his own struggles with med adherence and resistance. M.C. Mars brought us the truly unique perspective of a straight, tough-but-tender hip-hop cabbie living with HIV in San Francisco. "Anonymous" wrote of being a privileged white woman living secretly with HIV in the posh suburbs of New Jersey—only to finally "come out" on POZ's cover in 2006 as Regan Hofmann, the magazine's first HIV-positive editor-in-chief,

Clockwise from left: artwork by Frank Moore, female artists, people with AIDS

My Sisters' Keeper
BY SUZETTE MOSES-BURTON

A COLLECTION OF ART CREATED BY WOMEN INSPIRES AND UPLIFTS THE FEMALE SPIRIT.

SILENCE = DEATH

AIDS

Art of War
PWAs have made from AIDS some of the most powerful, provocative art of our time, and POZ has been honored to show it

Musto staked out the intersection between the epidemic and the glittery world of celebrity philanthropy. Several great writers also reported on HIV from far-flung parts of the world, including Austin Bunn in Thailand and Fariba Nawa in Iraq after the 2003 U.S.-led invasion.

In 2001, amid financial struggles, POZ nearly folded. When it got back on its feet, it was with a dramatically leaner editorial budget. For the past near-20 years, it's really the POZ staff, HIV positive and negative alike, that has stepped up and done much of the monthly and then—with the mid-2000s web revamp—daily heavy lifting of covering HIV/AIDS in all its manifestations.

For more than a decade, Laura Whitehorn, with help from Tim Horn, helmed the treatment section, covering nearly every important study and paying particular attention to often overlooked groups such as women and people in prison. Since 2013, Ben Ryan has been providing POZ's treatment coverage, digging into major developments of recent years, including pre-exposure prophylaxis (PrEP) and the Undetectable Equals Untransmittable (U=U) movement. Liz Highleyman, a long-term contributor, recently rejoined the fold as POZ's science editor.

Yours truly, combining my journalistic experience with my own journey as an HIV-positive person, took on issues such as treatment-resistant folks in the post-protease era and drug pricing. Cindra Feuer reported from abroad, particularly Uganda, whose HIV prevention strategy set a global model.

Kellee Terrell often covered HIV in the Black community, including deconstructing the oversimplified idea of Black men "on the down low"

a position she held until 2012. And in recent years, the impassioned My Fabulous Disease blogger Mark S. King has taken on thorny topics like enduring HIV stigma among gay men.

Of course, POZ has had more than its share of extraordinary HIV-negative writers, bringing with them a diverse array of expertise. Enid Vasquez, Lawrence Goodman, Catherine Hanssens, Patrick Califia, Liz Highleyman, Bob Lederer, Carmen Retzlaff, Anne-christine d'Adesky, Stacie Stukin, Esther Kaplan, Kai Wright, Rita Rubin and Jennifer Block all delved deep into knotty issues of HIV treatment and policy, from scheduled treatment interruptions (remember those?) and alternative therapies to HIV-positive moms having HIV-negative babies to harm reduction for people who use drugs and sex workers.

Hilary Beard and Tomika Anderson gave us deep dives into HIV in the Black community, especially on issues of doctor trust and high HIV rates among gay and bi men of color. Beloved Village Voice gossip columnist Michael

passing HIV from secret male lovers to wives and girlfriends. David Thorpe put his French fluency to good use to give us piercing profiles of Haitian activist Esther Boucicault and France's controversial, criminalization-happy Femmes Positives. HIV-positive LeRoy Whitfield (d. 2005), POZ's first Black staff editor, wove hard-nosed reporting with his own columns about refusing treatment of his own free will and approaching death. (That was a particularly painful chapter for the POZ staff.)

Walter Armstrong, POZ's politically and intellectually charged HIV-negative editor-in-chief from 1998 to 2005, wrote a thoughtful, usually provocative letter each month that often examined his own complicated efforts to stay negative. He also oversaw some of the magazine's most memorably outrageous covers, including a 2003 homage to pets that featured a distinctly unhappy-looking pooch in a wig, shades and pearls. The inevitable cover line? "Without our pets, we would wig out!"

Over Disclosure

A trick proposes, Dominic discloses, then calls the ho thing off

BY DOMINIC HAMILTON-LITTLE

Looking at his lips—lined by the gods with a slightly darker hue than his pure gingerbread complexion—I want to kiss them again. I've kissed them once. Briefly. On the dance floor of the nightclub we've just left. Instead, I smile at him, as those lips cradle the cold beer I've just cracked open for him, and launch into that brief routine that's become oh so familiar since I got my test result back at 11:30 a.m., September 9, 1993.

"Just so you know the score, Angelo, I play safe, and I'm HIV positive."

He splutters, sending a dribble of beer down his chin, and wiping it off with the back of one gorgeous hand, says, "Jesus Christ, that's fucked, man."

I am used to either the sweetly mundane—"Oh, I'm so sorry"—or the all-too-frequent, "That's okay, so am I." But what I hear this time, as he nearly chokes on his brew, pinches a nerve. Suddenly the evening is not progressing quite as it should.

"Well, I suppose you could say that," I attempt a smile. "I take it from your reaction that you haven't heard this very often."

"No, never." He pauses, and I wait in a ghastly, yawning chasm of eternity, wondering where he might be going. Believing, as a boy of the HIV brigade, that education is a burden I must carry, I am usually prepared to explain the intricacies of being fabulously positive. Any such pedagogic thoughts come crashing about my winsome head, however, with his next remark.

"Why didn't you tell me before we left the bar? I mean, then I could've…." He sounds petulant, almost churlish, as a child who has entered a candy store only to be told that all the candy had been sold.

"I beg your pardon?" My back stiffens.

"Why didn't you tell me right away?"

"Because. Because, I am not in the habit of disclosing such details whilst flirting on a dance floor and shaking my tight white rear end to Billie Ray Martin's 'Put Your Loving Arms

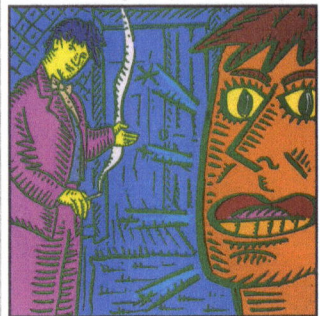

"I'm not ready to be your first openly positive lover."

Around Me,' and because I suppose it is my belief that if you have a problem with it, and suddenly don't want to fuck me, I'm not going to make it as easy for you as just walking away from me and up to the bar to order another cocktail from the stunning buffed bartender you like so well."

Listening to myself, I am mortified. I can't believe I've just said that. But bile is beginning to flow, and as my friends constantly say, I am moved by my spleen to utter the unutterable.

Sensing my ire, he turns his head away, picks an imaginary piece of lint off his beautifully cut woolen trousers, and says quietly, if somewhat desperately, "But I'm only 22. I don't want to die."

"None of us do. And though you will eventually, you

I suddenly don't want him and am simply too weary for the conversation and too bored to get angrier. "Listen sweetheart," I sigh, "there's plenty of places where you can pick up all the literature you could want on this, and you could even call the hotline for info. I'm a little tired, and I think it might be best for both of us if you left now." I get up and walk toward the door.

"Wait," he almost yells and grabs my arm. "Couldn't we perhaps, just, well, you know." He grins, and next thing I know his hand is rubbing my crotch. I feel stifled and awkward. This sudden remorse and change of heart confuses and annoys me. I mean, I wanted him. Yeah, since that first moment I saw him, before my pride was hurt. And I felt dirty. But now he wants me again.

No way. Pulling back, I open the door. "Look, sorry, but I'm just not ready to be your first openly HIV positive lover. It's not going to be that easy." He turns toward the door as I continue. "And please be safe, always. Just because you heard it first from me, don't imagine you haven't had sex with someone who is HIV positive and just didn't want to tell you—precisely because of how you've just reacted."

"You're something else, that's for sure. Take it easy." And with that he turns and walks out of my flat.

I am surprised at how much my hands are shaking as I light a cigarette and collapse onto the sofa. God, what a vile ending to the evening. As I remember dancing with him, and laughing, and kissing those lips, I realize with some relief that I don't want to kiss them anymore, not after what they'd said. ∎

ART: HARVEY REDDING FOR POZ

UNREALITY TV

With the TV cameras running, **River Huston** focuses on her fears—up close and too personal

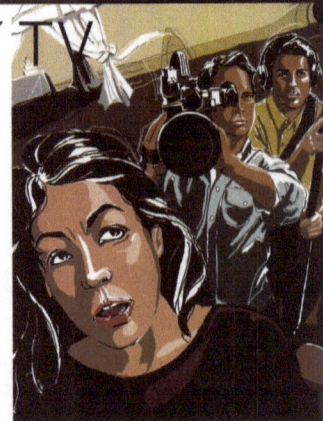

I HAVE BEEN LECTURING, WRITING AND PERforming a one-woman show about my life as a self-proclaimed HIV-enhanced goddess with a big mouth for the last 12 years. I weave messages of prevention, testing, self-respect—and, since moving to the country with my fiancé, my affinity for large farm equipment—into my talks. I'm pretty open about my life. So when Showtime asked to follow my fiancé and me around for a few weeks to make a documentary (as an openly positive/negative couple, we're newsworthy), I thought it would be one more chance to open some hearts and minds about AIDS.

It was much harder than I'd dreamed. The ever-present camera recorded tooth-brushing at night and prayers in the morning. Besides filming our life *verité*, the filmmakers interviewed each of us in depth. When they asked me if my honey had been tested—an obvious question, right?—I was surprised at how I shut down. Here I am, this educated educator, and I can't deal with my partner getting tested. I didn't even want to think about it. Next question. It made me realize that I had plowed my fear of infecting this man who is such a treasure to me deep beneath all my acceptance of HIV.

Now, unbeknownst to me, he had agreed to get tested, camera crew in tow. He'd wanted to for a while, but hadn't gotten around to it. Nothing like a film crew to help you keep appointments. One of his stipulations was that I couldn't know. He understood that my fear was illogical, and he thought the least stressful way to do it was to wait until after the test to tell me. So off they went, the crew pretending to follow him to work. The same charade unfolded when he went to get the results, which happened to be the day before our wedding.

When he returned from that second trip, we went to get the kilt he was going to wear for the wedding. He asked the cameras to stay behind so we could have some privacy (he respectfully knew I wouldn't want my meltdown filmed). I didn't think much of it until he revealed to me that he had been tested, received the results that morning and was negative.

I felt betrayed. When we drove up our long driveway and stepped into our house, the cameras were rolling and I

Here I am, an HIV educator, and I can't deal with my honey getting tested.

couldn't even look at the crew. I was furious with them—and with my partner for going behind my back. I walked out to the trees at the edge of our property. With my back to what felt like a crowd but was really only six, I sat in a chair and cried. He was negative, for God's sake—I couldn't understand why I was so distressed. After letting my irrational feelings fly for about 20 minutes, my head cleared and I saw what was really upsetting me. I'd done what many people do around this disease: I'd lived in denial because I was harboring deep-seated shame that I was diseased, untouchable and harmful to this man I love. I felt I wasn't deserving of the wonderful life we were having.

I felt like I'd uncovered an oozing, infected sore. I was stunned, disgusted—and relieved. The next day I married my honey in our backyard, walking down the red stone path he had just built, turning the corner to see all our loved ones standing in a field in front of the altar we had made together. The next week I went into therapy to help me keep that shame close to the surface so it could heal. ◦

ILLUSTRATIONS BY DAVID PFENDLER

Hofmann, Armstrong's successor, wrote the lion's share of features during her tenure, profiling fellow AIDS power players like amfAR's Kenneth Cole, the Black AIDS Institute's Phill Wilson and fledgling U.S. Senator Kirsten Gillibrand—and often supplementing old-fashioned multi-source reporting with stirring rhetorical calls to arms.

In 2012, Hofmann was succeeded by her deputy, a gay native New Yorker and former Marine, Oriol Gutierrez. The magazine's first HIV-positive editor-in-chief of color, he continued conducting his monthly Q&As with key HIV/AIDS activists and policymakers—and also began putting a special focus on the epidemic in the Latinx community, where HIV rates among gay and bi men had begun to rise.

Through all three editorships, managing editor Jennifer "Mama" Morton has not only kept this constant flow of editorial and artistic talent on track and on deadline but has also contributed to time- and labor-intensive "roundup" packages for the magazine's 10th, 15th, 20th and now 25th anniversary editions.

Then there are the myriad stories—large and small—cranked out by former and current staffers including Lucile Scott, Reed Vreeland, Alicia Green, Kate Ferguson, James Wortman, Joe Mejía, Trent Straube, Bob Ickes, Sally Chew, Nicole Joseph, Casey Halter and more. And we would be remiss not to mention the late Dennis Daniel (d. 2013), POZ's comptroller and human resources manager from day 1 and the magazine's resident expert on all matters show tunes and Broadway, especially regarding Liza Minnelli.

In recent years, the U.S. epidemic has concentrated stubbornly around Black folks, especially in the South and in gay, bi and trans communities. Those who have contributed cutting-edge reporting in this realm include Rod McCullom (who has also reported incisively about the epidemic in Puerto Rico), Mathew Rodriguez, Olivia Ford and Aundaray Guess, who has written movingly of his own experiences as an HIV-positive Black man trying to stick to his meds regimen—and receiving much-needed love and emotional nourishment from his dogs.

Fiction and poetry have been well represented in the magazine over the years as well, especially during the tenure of the lit-loving Armstrong. Poets Tory Dent (d. 2005) and Mary Bowman (d. 2019) wrote beautifully and heart-wrenchingly of life with the virus. Poet Jaime Manrique,

From left: columns by Dominic Hamilton-Little, River Huston, Shari Margolese, Mark Tuggle

ALTARED STATE

When I walk down the aisle this summer, will I look like I have HIV?

Love is in the air: I'm about to leave for the Caribbean to marry my partner of six years. We've planned an intimate seaside ceremony atop the black coral cliffs of Negril, Jamaica, near his parents' home. My fiancé and I are 42, but it's his first marriage, whereas I'm on my—call Jerry Springer—third. Yet I feel like a blushing first-timer. I daydream about the sun setting as we exchange the vows that will unite us and my 12-year-old son as a family. I have planned every detail: white roses and purple orchids for the bouquets. White-and-purple rose petals scattered on the aisle. Handmade candles flickering among orchid petals in the pool. After a traditional Jamaican wedding feast, we'll reggae and rock. And, ah, yes, my dress: it's strapless, mermaid-style...the dress! Wake up, Shari!

Reality scatters my fantasy. Although I've had HIV for 13 years, I've been spared what living with this disease can do to your body—until I dropped 20 pounds in just a few weeks during a bout with the flu (so much for the flu shot). My legs and arms thinned, my butt and breasts all but vanished, while my belly seemed to swell. It turned out that underneath my middle-age plumpness, I had the typical signs of lipodystrophy.

Now that my shirts are baggy and my pants sag, my skateboarding son thinks I look "stylin'." As much as I appreciate the support, what will my 30 wedding guests say about my weight change? Will they ask about my health? Will I look ill in my photo albums? Am I being shallow and vain?

I have never obsessed over my looks. I've long since lost the beauty-queen bod I strutted in the 1982 Miss Canada pageant. Indeed, my extra bulk has served as an "insurance policy" to be cashed in if I got sick. Now, my insurance has expired, and when I look in the mirror, I no longer feel healthy, curved, sexy—but like a pregnant Kate Moss. My man, who dreams of a princess bride, has noticed. I was making cookies when he grabbed my butt and asked "What happened to the junk in the trunk?" I hoped it was a compliment. Then he added, "I hope those cookies are for you—you could use a few pounds." I was mortified. How would he react if I got PCP or something worse? Sometimes I feel selfish asking him to commit to a future that could include a sickly looking

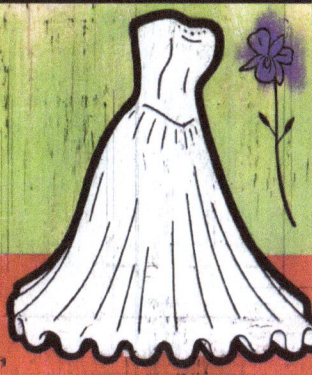

"What's your weight-loss secret?" his cousins asked.

wife instead of the slightly rounded goddess he signed up for.

Prewedding festivities have also put me under the microscope. His cousins threw me a lingerie shower. After a few glasses of wine, they persuaded me to model the gifts. Everyone noticed I'd lost weight, but, to my shock, they all thought I looked fabulous. "What's your secret?" they demanded. I'd forgotten that weight loss was an achievement in the HIV negative world. His family doesn't know my status, so I replied, "Ah, you know, drink lots of water, walk the dog. No real secret." I had a secret, all right—but one I wasn't willing to share.

My doc helped put things in perspective. Although concerned, she explained that anyone can lose 20 pounds with a bad case of the flu. She added that since I switched to a combo of Kaletra and Combivir last summer, my CD4s have bounced from 400 to 780 and my viral load has gone from over 100,000 to undetectable.

Assured that I wasn't about to die anytime soon, I went to pick up my dress: A strapless, mermaid-style "hoochie mama" gown in white net reminiscent of Marilyn Monroe's in Diamonds Are a Girl's Best Friend. The salon owner helped me find the right underwear to cinch my waist and push up my breasts and added a bustle to create a butt! Even I have to admit I looked amazing. I'm still anxious about a possible future of sunken cheeks (facial and otherwise) and scrawny arms, but at least I won't have to face it alone. I am marrying the love of my life. I'll be his princess bride. ◼

Shari Margolese was recently awarded the Golden Jubilee Medal of Queen Elizabeth II for her AIDS activism.

V I E W S

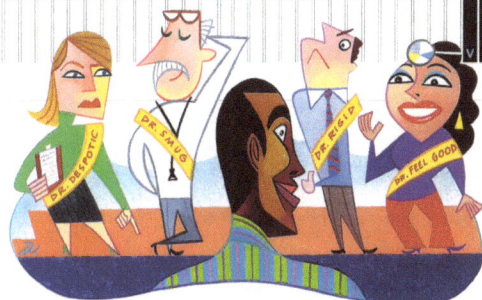

Doctor Feel Good

MARK TUGGLE LANDS THE TOUGH BUT TENDER PHYSICIAN OF HIS DREAMS

The first time I went to my current doctor's office, I was as anxious and excited as a teenager waiting for a blind date to ring the doorbell. She was a highly recommended AIDS specialist, and, despite eight doctors in as many years. I was still optimistic about finding "the One." After a short wait, the nurse led me to an office and left, closing the door behind her. When the door opened, I smiled and said, "Are you going to take care of me?" My new doctor touched my shoulder and gently replied, "Only if you let me, dear."

And then I exhaled.

Finding the right physician is as daunting a task as finding the right lover. Every person with HIV brings their unique personality to the examining room—and so does each doctor. I'm a warm, gentle, passionate, 44-year-old same-gender-loving man of African descent. I can also be arrogant and unyielding—I was born with an attitude. MDs can be difficult, too: Many forget just who is living with HIV and react with horror if you miss taking a pill. That's a shame because HIV docs are more than medical professionals. They are our nutritionists, safer-sex gurus, therapists and, if we're lucky, friends.

I was diagnosed in the winter of '94. Though I was asymptomatic, I became terrified and obsessed with death—like Tupac and Biggie, but for a different reason. My first physician was, like me, a strong believer in holistic health. Yet he never asked me how I felt about AIDS. So I was afraid to be honest with him about the difficulties of my life: I was newly in recovery, frightened of HIV meds and uncomfortable talking about my sexual behavior.

When I checked in one afternoon, the receptionist casually informed me that the facility no longer employed him. Damn—no letter, no phone call, nothing. I felt like a dumped

My doc is warm, caring— and don't take no shit from me.

boyfriend. The staff dutifully referred me to a same-gender-loving black female doc, which gave me hope that we might connect. But when I shared my fears around taking meds, she barked, in front of three other physicians, "Well, don't call me when you end up in the emergency room."

I felt like Rodney Dangerfield.

By '97, I was feeling better about myself: I'd added acupuncture, workouts, prayer, meditation and vitamins to my health regimen. My physician at the time, though, was cold and distant. I dreaded each visit. He rushed examinations and talked too fast. I'd enter confident and leave confused.

Such experiences make me realize how blessed I am to have my present doc. That she's fiftysomething and Latina puts me at ease. She's also warm, caring—and don't take no shit from me. When I told her I'd had unprotected sex with a positive partner, she said, "Do you love him enough to die for him?" She was right: The risk of reinfection or an STD wasn't worth it.

A few years ago, right around the time I found my doc, I started having serious health issues: night sweats, pneumonia, weight loss, skin problems. Her unwavering support and assurances that others have recovered from similar illnesses have made all the difference. My doc affirms the value of my ongoing healing and empowerment and helps me to be a person with HIV who is joyous and free.

During a recent visit, she said something that made me certain she was Dr. Right: "Mark, you've made tremendous progress. You're so serene now. When we began working together, you were such a bitch." I laughed so hard my stomach was in knots. The truth hurts—and it sets you free.

---

playwright Paula Vogel and novelists Mary Gaitskill, Andrew Holleran, Edmund White and Sarah Schulman have all appeared in these pages.

Oh, and did we mention art, design and photography? From those very first issues featuring the witty caricatures of Robert Risko and the gorgeous cover portraits of Greg Gorman, POZ—often in conjunction with the group Visual AIDS, whose board includes POZ's Jennifer Morton—has filled its pages with stunning images from the likes of artists including Barton Lidicé Beneš (d. 2012), Frank Moore (d. 2002), Ben Cuevas and the brilliant and funny collagist Tom Cocotos and such lens masters as Bill Bytsura, Arlene Gottfried (d. 2017), Kristen Ashburn and Spencer Tunick, who famously, for POZ's 10th anniversary cover, created an installation of scores of buck-naked HIV-positive folks. (The chilly early morning setting was the late, great New York diner Florent, named after its openly HIV-positive French proprietor, Florent Morellet, who provided the POZ family with a virtual canteen for many years.) In recent years, the talented Bill Wadman has taken countless luminous photos of POZ's story subjects, positive and negative alike.

Magazine making takes more than art, of course. Design and production are essential. The pages of POZ owe their visual appeal to the art department—from POZ's first art director J.C. Suarès (d. 2013) to its current art director, Doriot Kim, as well as art production manager Michael Halliday, POZ's longest-serving staff member.

There is just one more set of POZ contributors (aside from the business folks) without whom the magazine could not have existed, and that is the literally thousands of people, in the United States and abroad, who were not afraid to speak openly about their lives with HIV and show their faces in the pages of POZ to provide comfort, courage and wisdom to readers, to break down the stigma that thrives on silence and invisibility, to make us laugh, cry, relate and empathize.

From HIV duo Michelle Lopez and her adorable daughter Raven to equally bite-size cover girl Hydeia Broadbent, from Larry Kramer to Phill Wilson to Hamilton superstar Javier Muñoz, and from '80s pop star Sherri Lewis to trans pioneers Chloe Dzubilo (d. 2011) and Cecilia Chung, the folks in the pages of POZ's first quarter-century prove that, time and again, people living with HIV and their allies have always pushed back against the forces of sickness, stigma and discrimination with a great collective cry of defiance, justice and joy. ◼

25
Years of Personal Stories

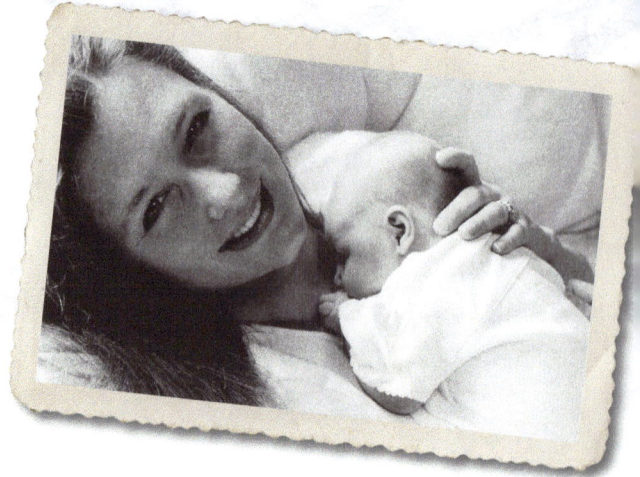

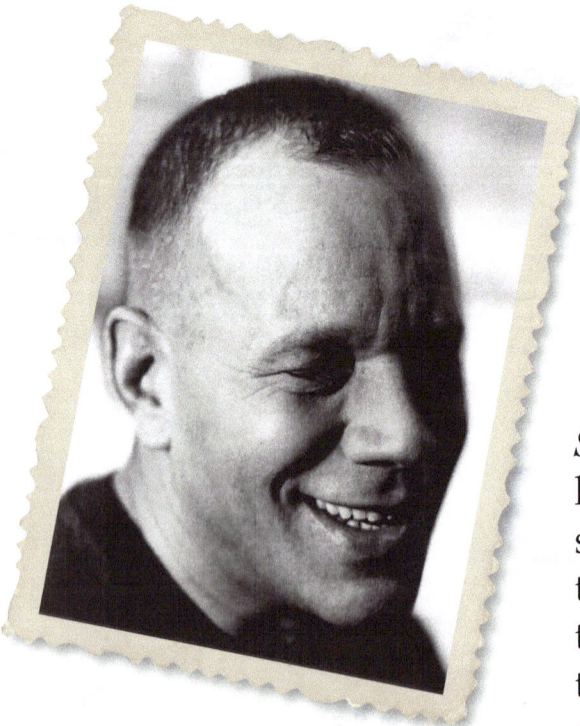

AMPLIFYING THE VOICES OF PEOPLE ON THE FRONT LINES OF THE FIGHT AGAINST HIV

BY ALICIA GREEN

Since 1994, POZ has featured countless people living with HIV in its pages. The subjects in these stories—everyone from everyday people who beat the odds to headline-grabbing advocates who spoke truth to power—have inspired readers throughout the country to take action, be resilient and remain optimistic even in dark times.

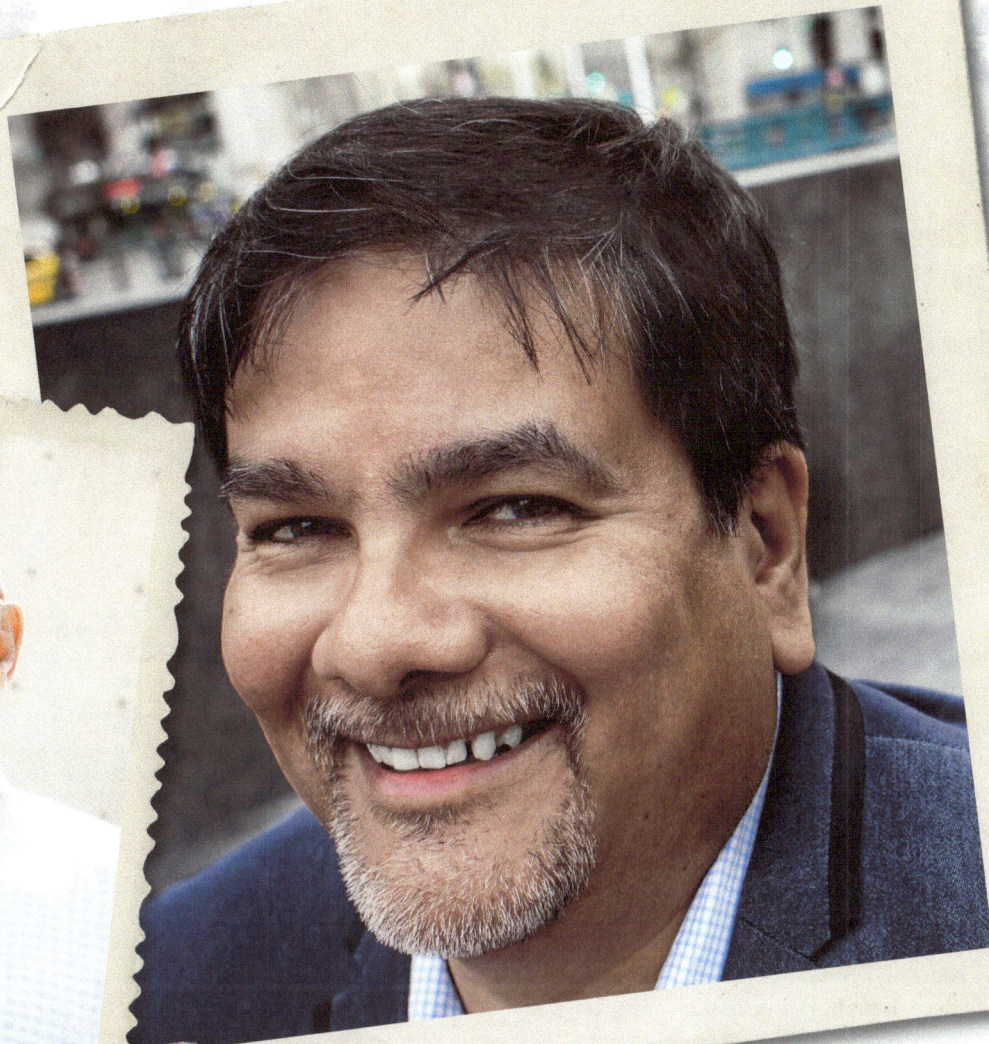

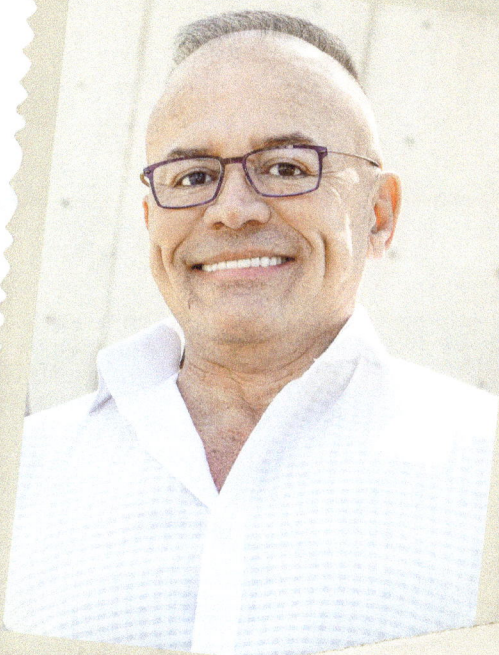

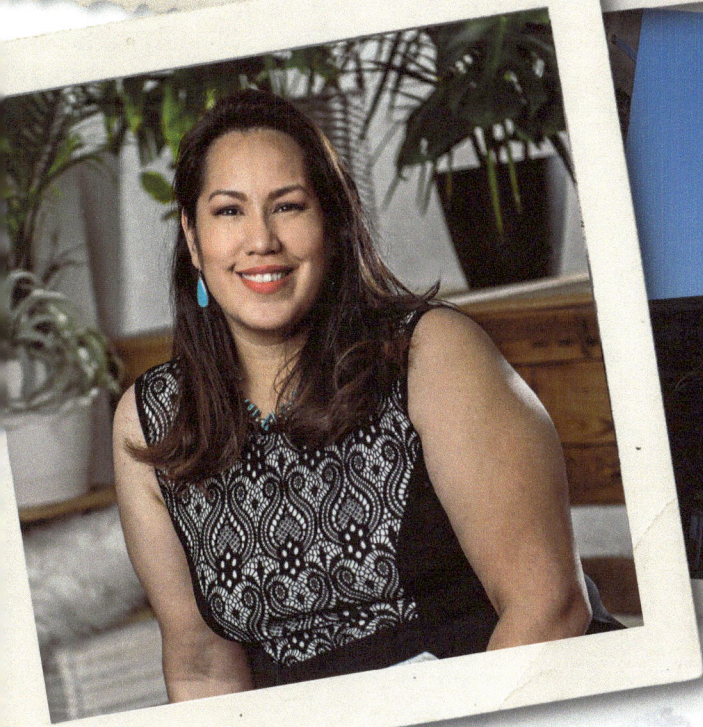

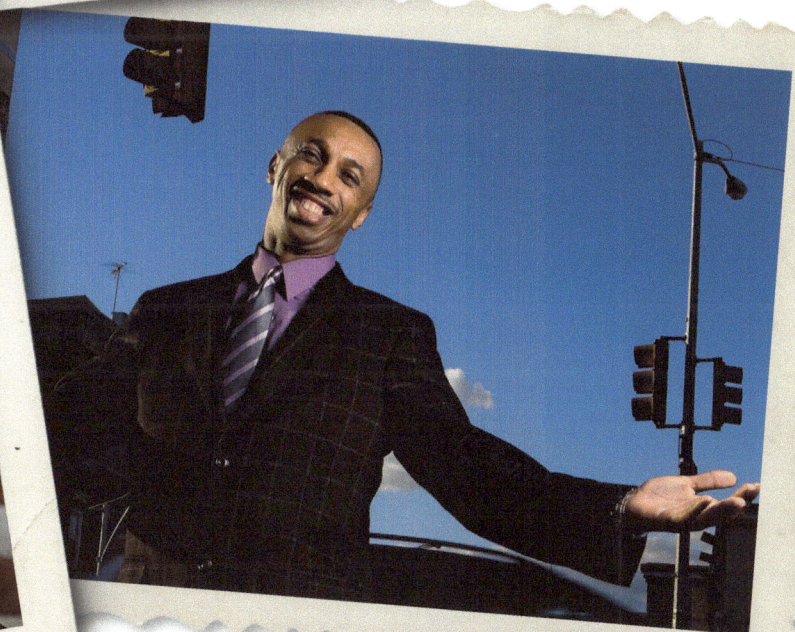

"POZ was a nexus for the PLHIV [people living with HIV] self-empowerment movement," said founder Sean Strub in an interview for the 25th anniversary issue.

"I'm really proud of the people we featured in the magazine who were previously unknown to a large audience," he said. "We consciously sought out people living with HIV doing great work and intentionally shined a spotlight on them as a strategy to amplify their voices and bring attention and resources to their work."

The folks highlighted here represent just a tiny fraction of the personal stories POZ has shared over the years. However, they serve as examples of the many diverse groups affected by HIV, including long-term survivors, transgender people, women, Latinos and African Americans. These are their stories.

Fred Bingham

In 1981, when Bingham was diagnosed with AIDS, he changed his lifestyle. He experimented with herbs, stopped using street drugs and started taking Antabuse to combat his alcohol use disorder.

He also took massive amounts of antioxidants to restore sulfur-containing amino acids, and he learned everything he could about AIDS.

In 1987, AZT became the first drug approved for the treatment of HIV. However, its side effects were so terrible that many of those who took it stopped using it altogether. Like many people back then, Bingham relied instead on alternative treatments to fight the disease.

But in 1989, the professional horticulturist started using drugs and alcohol again and abandoned his health regimen. He experienced severe thrush and neuropathy, weight loss and stress. He was also diagnosed with dementia and wound up in the hospital with a CD4 count of 39.

Bingham requested AZT to help treat the neuropathy that was affecting his body (even though now we know AZT causes neuropathy) but soon stopped taking the medication because of its toxicity. That's when he began to develop his own long-term intervention to manage his AIDS.

Once he got back on track, doctors were stunned to find that Bingham had reversed his condition. In 1994, Bingham, who then had a CD4 count of about 900, told POZ, "Technically, I'm in remission." He also believed that "the one-drug, one-bug, one-million-dollar mentality [was] not serving people with HIV and AIDS very well."

In response, Bingham founded Direct AIDS Alternative Information Resources, a nonprofit group that promoted self-empowered healing from HIV and its related illnesses. He operated it from his apartment. It was this do-it-yourself advocacy that the HIV community best remembered when he died in 2015.

Veronika Cauley

A Black HIV and transgender activist from San Francisco, Cauley was determined to make the health care system work for the transgender community.

Since the start of the epidemic, transgender people have had to fight to make their voices heard. In 1999, POZ wrote its first extensive story on this population. The article highlighted alarming HIV rates in San Francisco among transgender African-American women as well as discrimination and other barriers to care faced by people of trans experience.

The article also shone a light on Cauley, who began her transition in 1978 after leaving the Navy. She turned to sex work before becoming addicted to crack cocaine and getting arrested while living in New York City.

Cauley then fled to Indiana, where at the local Veterans Administration hospital she learned she had HIV—and doctors told her she had only five years to live. But Cauley continues to outlast her presumed expiration date.

After relocating to San Francisco, she lobbied to be appointed to the city's veterans affairs (VA) commission to update HIV treatments in VA hospitals.

In 2018, Cauley—now Veronika Fimbres—hoped to become California's first African-American transgender governor as a write-in candidate for the Green Party.

As she told POZ 25 years ago: "I have hope for the future— that they will find a cure, that transgenders will no longer

POZ coverage, clockwise from left: Veronika Cauley, Dawn Averitt, Stacy Latimer

Love Me GENDER

Transgendered people with HIV are making the system work for them

BY PAT CALIFIA

THE FIRST THING VERONIKA CAULEY does when we meet on a rainy Saturday afternoon at the Lyon-Martin Women's Health Services clinic in San Francisco is define her terms: She prefers the label *transgendered*, or *TG*, to *transsexual*.

"As I experienced my femaleness for the first time, I REMINDED MYSELF OF MARLO THOMAS in *That Girl* twirling around downtown."

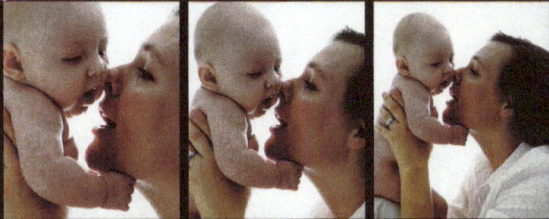

Baby Love

ONCE, HAVING HIV DASHED HOPES OF MOTHERHOOD—GIVING YOUR BABY THE VIRUS OR LEAVING HER AN ORPHAN WAS UNTHINKABLE. BUT WITH NEAR-PERFECT PREVENTION AND LONG, HEALTHY LIVES, WOMEN WITH HIV ARE MAKING A DREAM DEFERRED COME TRUE

BY STACIE STUKIN

WHAT A GIRL!: DAWN AVERITT, 33, BRINGS DAUGHTER MADDY (8 POUNDS, 5 OUNCES) INTO THE WORLD, JOINING THE HIVer BABY BOOM

"There has been a child inside me waiting to come into this world for as long as I can remember. She has shown up in my dreams and been part of my psyche. Have you ever wanted something so deeply that you could feel it coursing through your veins and permeating every fiber of your being? If you have, then you know." HIVer Dawn Averitt wrote in a recent essay tellingly subtitled "Tough Choices…and the Right to Choose" in the *Journal of the Association of Nurses and AIDS Care*.

Averitt, a high-profile AIDS activist who lives in Asheville, North Carolina, tested positive in 1988 at age 19. Her first tentative inquiries about the possibility of ever having a child were met with grim statistics—she had a 70 to 100 percent chance of infecting her baby—and comments such as "Only consider it if you're a homicidal maniac." This was, of course, before HAART and undetectable viral loads, before tests to measure virus in the blood, before scientists even knew how HIV is passed from mother to child. Positive women faced a Sophie's choice—either abort the fetus or gamble with your baby's life.

Today, federal researchers trumpet the reduction of perinatal (prebirth) HIV transmission as the biggest success story of the epidemic. Studies show that babies are mostly infected during childbirth or breast-feeding, and that a combination of effective HAART, good health care and bottle-feeding guarantees that 99 out of every 100 HIVers can become mothers with virtually no risk to their baby. So just as the Pill once revolutionized women's sexual lives, HIV meds are radically changing what it means to have HIV, extending not only life expectancy but life expectations. The time is ripe for a baby boom among the HIV parenting set. And with women making up almost a third of the estimated 900,000 HIVers in the U.S., the trend could be tremendous.

be devalued. Because I think it's the world's diversity that makes it a better place."

Dawn Averitt

When Averitt was diagnosed with HIV in 1988 at age 19, she didn't think motherhood would be an option for her. She recalled coming across a statistic proclaiming that a pregnant woman with HIV had a 70% to 100% chance of transmitting the virus to her baby. But Averitt really wanted to be a mother.

Then, in 1996, the advent of effective antiretroviral (ARV) therapy for HIV meant that a mom with the virus no longer had to fear that her children would be orphaned in the near future. But was it safe to give birth? Averitt worried that the meds would be harmful to a fetus.

The reassuring answer to Averitt's question came in the form of a 2001 study that revealed that taking ARVs during the first trimester of pregnancy did not increase the risk for birth defects. Further research showed that HIV treatment combined with good health care and bottle-feeding guaranteed that 99 out of every 100 women with HIV could become mothers with virtually no risk to their baby.

So Averitt decided to become a mother. In June 2002, she and her husband welcomed an HIV-negative daughter, Maddy, into the world. Averitt and Maddy graced the cover of POZ's December 2002 issue. That same year, Averitt founded The Well Project, a nonprofit that works to improve the lives of women living with HIV.

For long-term survivors, Averitt has this bit of advice: "Integrate HIV into your life. If you let HIV be a tumor, an invader, a growth, then the burden is too heavy. Once it is a part of your life (and not the sum total of your life), HIV becomes more manageable."

The Reverend Stacy Latimer

Latimer, one of our 2007 cover subjects, is an HIV-positive minister and military vet who has relationships with men.

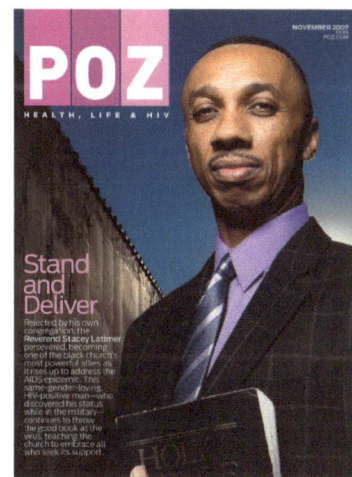

The South Carolina native grew up in a religious family and had known from childhood that he was attracted to men. He kept this hidden throughout his adolescence, causing him much pain.

In 1987, while enlisted in the Army, Latimer learned he was HIV positive via a letter from the Red Cross about a blood donation he'd made. After sharing his diagnosis with a commanding officer, he was sent to Walter Reed Medical Center in Washington, DC, which housed servicemen with HIV in a special ward.

Latimer spent so much of his time at the hospital comforting those who were critically ill and had been abandoned that patients assumed he was a volunteer.

However, Latimer still had his own demons to face. Struggling to process his HIV diagnosis, he turned to drugs and alcohol to help him cope. But Latimer says God came to him one night and showed him his purpose. He soon quit drugs and studied to become a religious leader.

Latimer went on to establish his own AIDS ministry and work closely with other pastors and faith leaders who have tested positive for the virus. Most important, he has traveled to Black churches and helped take on the difficult topic of HIV in their own congregations. He accomplishes this by sharing his own testimony and inspiring others to do the same.

"Our stories, told with sincerity and integrity, carry the power to heal," he told POZ. "They share wisdom, usher in peace and impart strength."

Antonio Muñoz

Muñoz was diagnosed with HIV in 2008. At the time, he was about a year into his job at The Manhattan Club, a boutique hotel in New York City, and didn't think he needed to disclose his status.

Between 2007 and 2011, Muñoz was such a model employee that he received the Exemplary Manager Award, several raises and positive evaluations from supervisors.

As his health declined, Muñoz's doctor prescribed Sustiva, a drug known to cause drowsiness. This concerned Muñoz, who knew he could no longer work nights at the hotel. He asked for a shift change and submitted a doctor's note explaining his health problems but was initially denied. Eventually, he was switched to a day shift.

But soon, the hotel put Muñoz back on the night shift. When he complained about it to human resources, his supervisors retaliated against him. Then, in 2011, after someone made an anonymous complaint about him, he was fired from his job.

Muñoz filed a lawsuit against The Manhattan Club for discrimination. In its counterargument, the hotel characterized Muñoz as a lazy complainer who didn't do his job. Muñoz rejected that idea and said he was only trying to take care of his health.

In April 2013, a jury ruled in his favor in federal court. Muñoz was awarded $500,000 for wrongful termination as a result of HIV discrimination.

But it was never just about the money for Muñoz. It was about telling his story and being heard. As he told POZ readers in 2014: "You have to have determination to believe in yourself."

Shana Cozad

A member of the Kiowa tribe in Oklahoma, Cozad has lived with HIV for more than two decades and is one of the first Native American women to speak openly about her HIV status. She is also one of nearly 4,000 American Indians and Alaska Natives estimated to be living with the virus.

While in college, Cozad contracted the virus from her boyfriend, who was only her second sexual partner. But it wasn't until their breakup that he admitted to having AIDS. She didn't believe him and assumed it was just a desperate ploy to keep them together.

A friend eventually convinced Cozad to get tested. It took

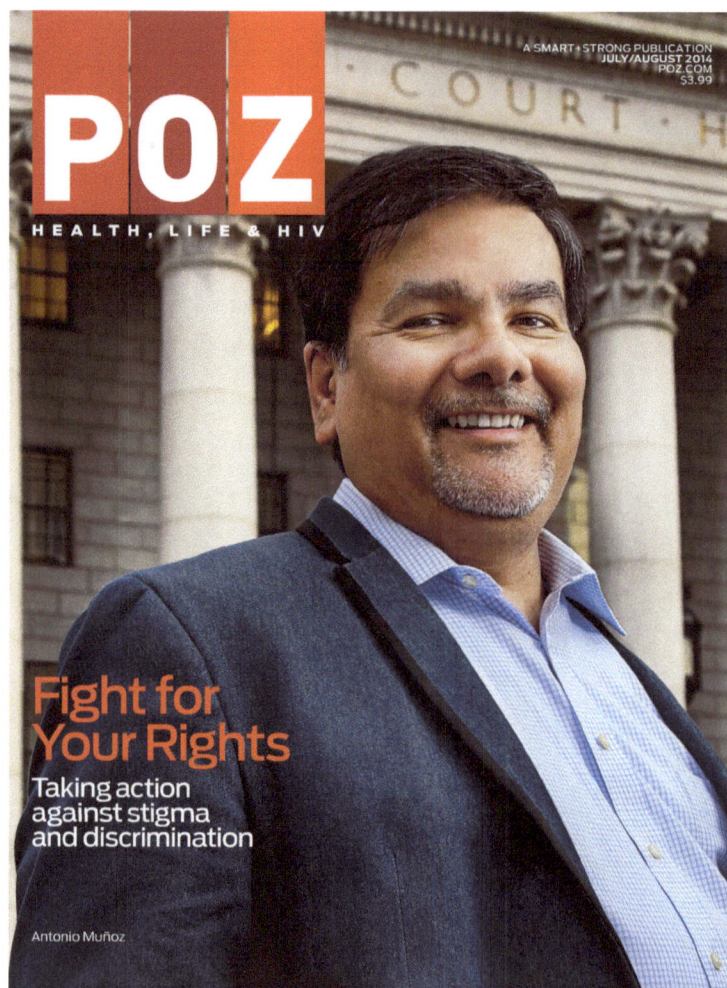

A SMART + STRONG PUBLICATION
JULY/AUGUST 2014
POZ.COM
$3.99

POZ
HEALTH, LIFE & HIV

Fight for Your Rights
Taking action against stigma and discrimination

Antonio Muñoz

Coverage by POZ, from left: Antonio Muñoz, Shana Cozad, Nelson Vergel

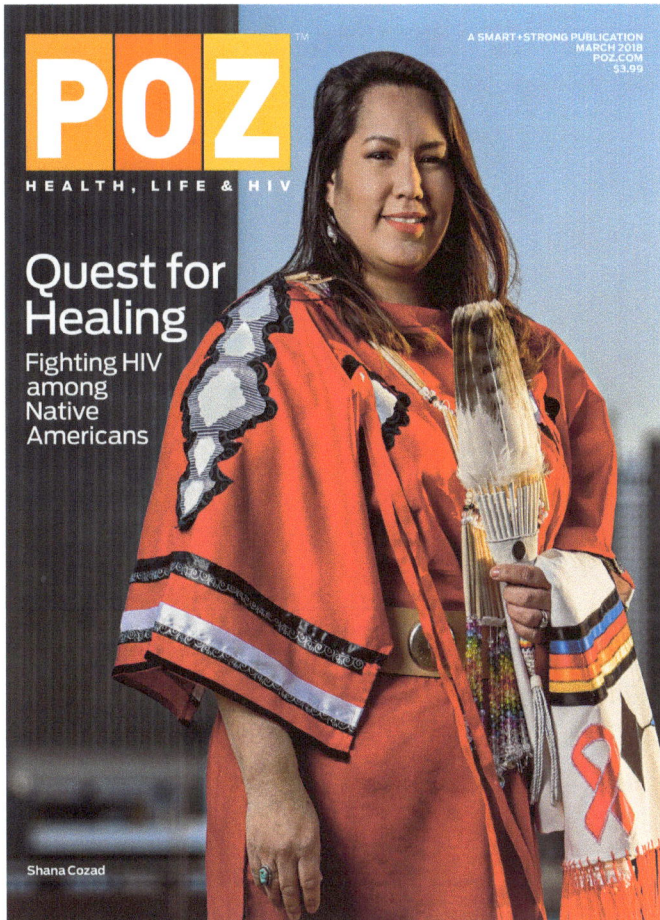

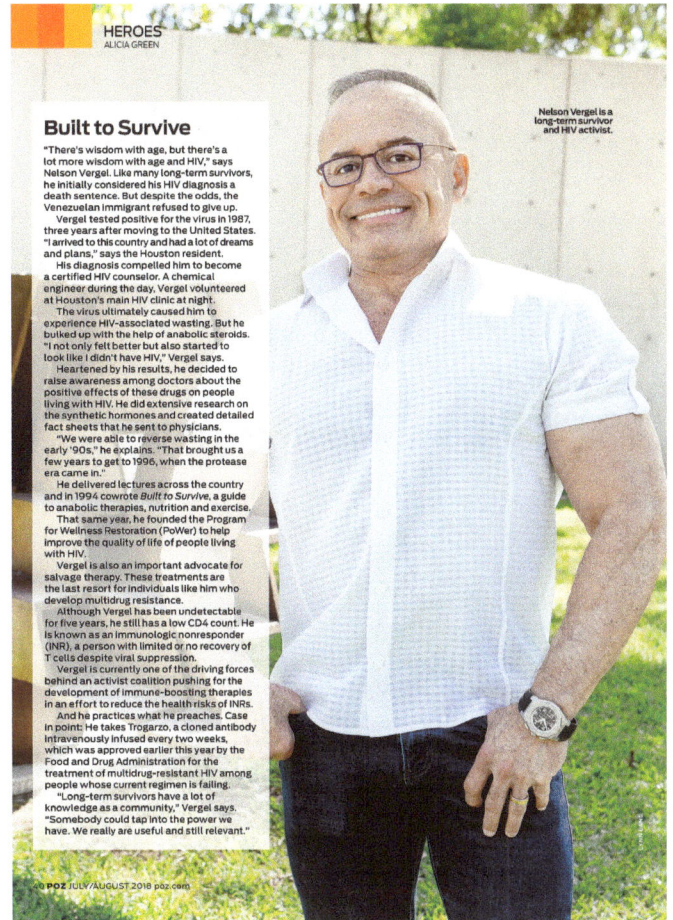

three positive test results for Cozad to finally accept her diagnosis. Unfortunately, she also learned that her CD4 count was 189 and she was living with AIDS despite feeling fine.

Following her diagnosis, she turned to her tribal elders for help. They guided her through traditional healing ceremonies and overnight rites that lasted 12 to 15 hours. These ceremonies, Cozad said, helped release her anger at HIV.

Today, Cozad's virus is undetectable. For this, she credits not only her antiretroviral medication but also her spiritual advisers, who taught her how to approach the disease and her body in a positive manner. In 2018, she told POZ, "HIV is a teacher for me. It has transformed my life. It has humbled me. I don't feel cured, but I feel healed because I'm at peace with this disease."

Nelson Vergel

When Vergel immigrated to the United States from Venezuela in 1984, he had a lot of dreams and plans. But they were all cut short when he tested positive for HIV just three years later. He considered his diagnosis a death sentence.

But Vergel never gave up. Instead, he told POZ in 2018, he became a certified HIV counselor who worked as a chemical engineer during the day and as a volunteer at a local clinic at night.

The virus caused Vergel to experience HIV-associated wasting, so he turned to anabolic steroids to help him regain weight. His success led him to advocate for these drugs for people living with HIV. In 1994, he cowrote *Built to Survive*, a guide to anabolic therapies, nutrition and exercise, and founded the Program for Wellness Restoration (PoWer) to help improve the quality of life for those with HIV.

When Vergel's HIV became resistant to multiple drug therapies, he campaigned for salvage therapy—the development of entirely new meds—as a last resort for those like him. Luckily, he began to take Trogarzo, which was approved by the Food and Drug Administration in 2018 for the treatment of multidrug-resistant HIV among people whose current regimen is failing.

Since 2013, Vergel has had an undetectable viral load. But he still has a low CD4 count. This has prompted him to join an activist coalition that pushes for the development of immune-boosting therapies to reduce health risks for immunologic nonresponders, or people with limited or no recovery of CD4s despite viral suppression.

"Long-term survivors have a lot of knowledge as a community," Vergel shared with POZ in 2018. "Somebody could tap into the power we have. We really are useful and still relevant." ■

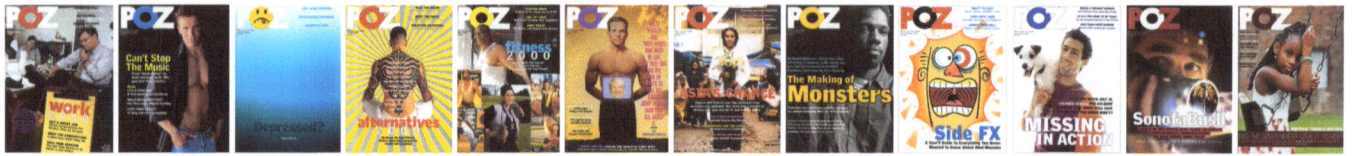

THE YEAR IN POZ

2000

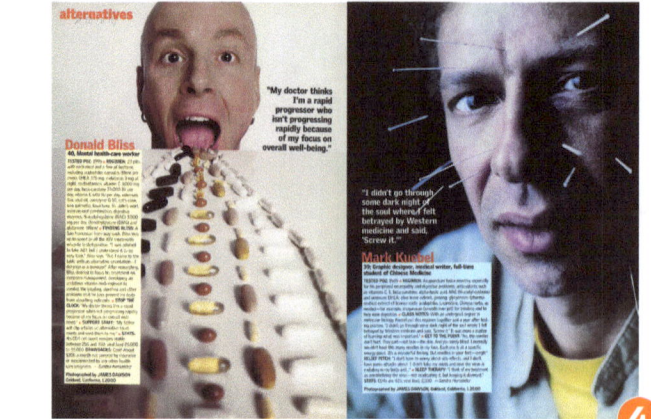

January

COVER: A profile of New York State Senator Tom Duane, the first openly HIV-positive elected official in the country. **INSIDE:** A look at the 25 friendliest companies for people living with AIDS; artist Valerie Caris uses her body for money and art—and a source of healing (1). **PLUS:** New testing options for drug resistance.

April

COVER: Seven people living with HIV explain why they are choosing alternative therapies (4). **INSIDE:** POZ separates the wheatgrass from the chaff in today's high-risk, low-regulation supplements market; the FDA's policy of banning gay men from donating blood comes under new fire. **PLUS:** Is Celia Farber the most dangerous AIDS reporter?

February

COVER: Pop star Paul "Boom Boom" Lekakis takes us back to his room for a juicy tell-all about life in—and out—of the strobe-lit closet. **INSIDE:** Eight feel-good yoga postures to ease the pain and stress of HIV; animal rights activists and AIDS activists lock horns over animal testing (2). **PLUS:** Photographer William Gedney finds fame after death.

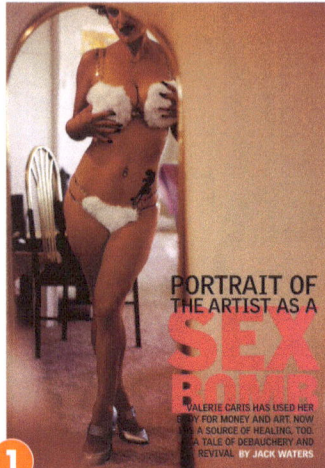

May

COVER: Exercise gives your health a boost by protecting your immune system and improving your appetite, energy and mood. **INSIDE:** How the fight for research funding is playing out in the disease wars (5); are fusion inhibitors the next big thing, or will their development fizzle out? **PLUS:** John Raynard's photo essay of Russians who inject drugs spotlights the country's growing HIV epidemic.

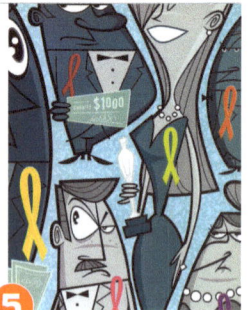

March

COVER: Emily Carter shares an insider's account of a battle on two fronts—HIV and clinical depression (3). **INSIDE:** Are microbicides the next big thing in HIV prevention? **PLUS:** Choreographers Chris Ramos and Fay Simpson perform bold new works about the risks and rewards of coming out as HIV positive.

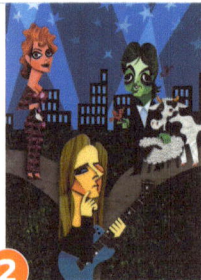

June

COVER: Jerry Falwell's gay cousin comes out of the HIV closet and asks for some Christian compassion (6). **INSIDE:** Kiss lipodystrophy's lumps, lines and puppet faces goodbye with plastic surgery. **PLUS:** Traveling while living with HIV takes some pre-vacation planning.

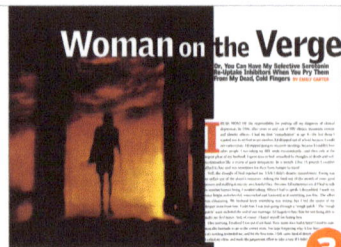

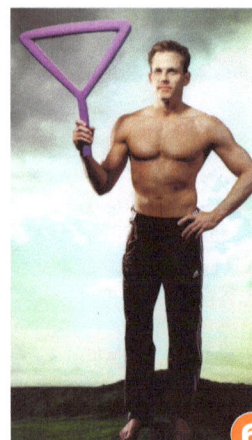

July

COVER: From Nepal to the Philippines, hear the voices from Asia's exploding HIV epidemic. **INSIDE:** Indonesia's designer-activist Suzana Murni on coming out as HIV positive (**7**); Ayurveda's ancient remedies attract Indians living with HIV as well as AIDS researchers. **PLUS:** A volunteer for Doctors Without Borders working in Cambodia shares her AIDS outreach photo diary.

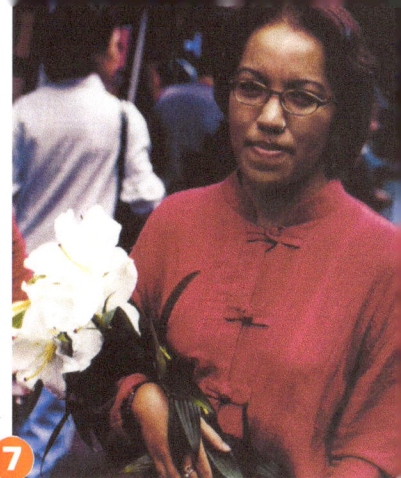

August

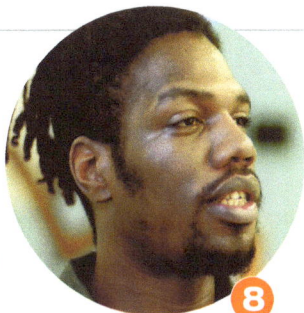

COVER: "AIDS monster" Nushawn Williams transmitted HIV to seven girls after testing positive, but he claims he never knew his status (**8**). **INSIDE:** The first national index of HIV criminalization cases; anal and cervical cancer are killer threats, which is why early Pap screenings are key. **PLUS:** Hot summer reads from Anne-christine d'Adesky, Philip Huang, Jaime Manrique and Ernesto Quiñonez.

September

COVER: A user's guide to everything you wanted to know about the side effects of HIV meds (**9**). **INSIDE:** A list of Congress's biggest AIDS foes (and friends) on the ballot; *Men Like Us: The GMHC Complete Guide to Gay Men's Sexual, Physical and Emotional Well-Being* covers everything from AIDS to aging to anal sex. **PLUS:** Cleve Jones, creator of the AIDS Memorial Quilt, is having a midlife crisis.

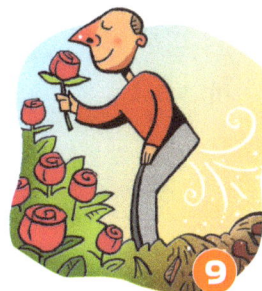

October

COVER: Remembering Stephen Gendin, the AIDS activist and HIV guinea pig who put his body on the line testing treatment theories, experimental drugs and new combinations (**10**). **INSIDE:** Behind the scenes of the 13th International AIDS Conference in Durban, South Africa. **PLUS:** Mark Schoofs's eight-part series on AIDS in Africa for The Village Voice wins the Pulitzer Prize for international reporting.

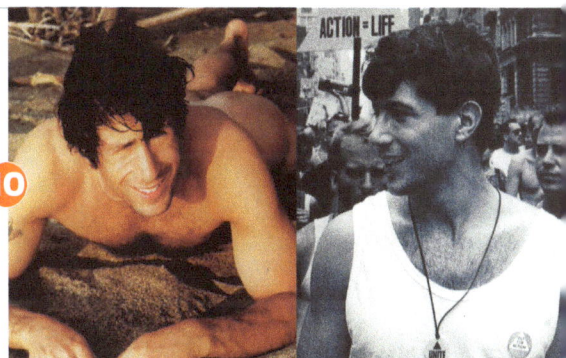

November

COVER: An HIV voting guide on the records and rhetoric of presidential candidates Gore, Bush, Nader and Buchanan. **INSIDE:** Donna Minkowitz travels to Philadelphia for the Republican convention; figure skater Rudy Galindo's glide from trailer park to trophies to HIV champ (**11**). **PLUS:** The secret life of syphilis, another STI shrouded in stigma.

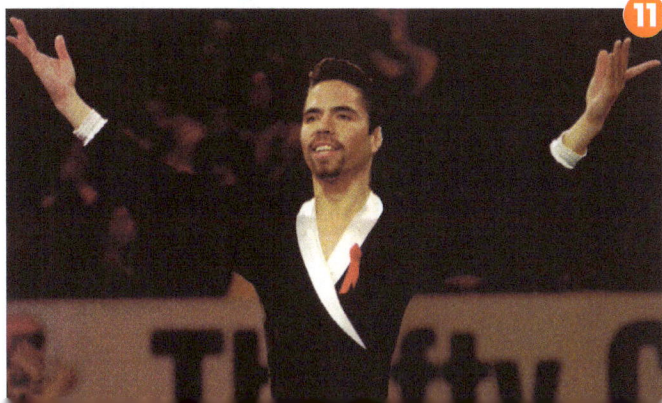

December

COVER: One out of four African Americans believe AIDS is a plot to eliminate the Black community (**12**). **INSIDE:** The year's biggest underreported HIV-related stories and scandals; from painkillers to medical marijuana, HIV medications can pose a tough challenge for people in recovery. **PLUS:** Why West Hollywood is in a tizzy over the Safer Sex City Act, which would make condom bowls a must in bars.

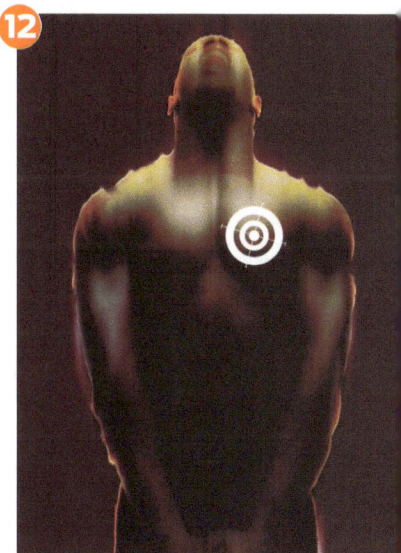

2001

January

COVER: It's time to make finding a cure the primary goal of treatment activism (1). **INSIDE:** A survey of so-called cures from the past; more and more people with HIV are contending with lymphoma; a chat with *Tales of the City*'s Armistead Maupin about his latest novel, *The Night Listener*. **PLUS:** A biography of film-maker Derek Jarman, who died of AIDS-related causes.

February/March

COVER: Six people living with HIV on how AIDS, addiction and other dark nights launched them on radically different spiritual journeys. **INSIDE:** Organized religion's 20-year love-hate relationship with people with AIDS; a couple's account of their life-and-death struggle for a liver transplant (2). **PLUS:** The fight to renew an HIV drug.

April

COVER: A special report examines the economics of AIDS (3). **INSIDE:** How to live large on small change, as told by three supersavers with HIV; does big pharma prioritize profit over people living with HIV? **PLUS:** Departed AIDS Action head Jamie Fox dishes to Doug Ireland on why he resigned.

May

COVER: Nearly one third of urban Black gay men in their 20s have HIV. One 21-year-old shares his story. **INSIDE:** An up-to-the-minute guide on when to start opportunistic infection prevention; South African activists with HIV are getting meds to people with AIDS by any means necessary (4). **PLUS:** Health officials flip-flop on antiretroviral treatment guidelines.

June

COVER: Three long-termers share lessons on how to tough it out when HIV kicks your butt year after year. **INSIDE:** Michael Gottlieb, MD, authored the first report on AIDS and has been at the bedside of PWAs ever since; Liz Murray wasn't born with HIV, but, with two positive parents, she grew up with it (5). **PLUS:** AIDS drug counterfeiting hits the United States.

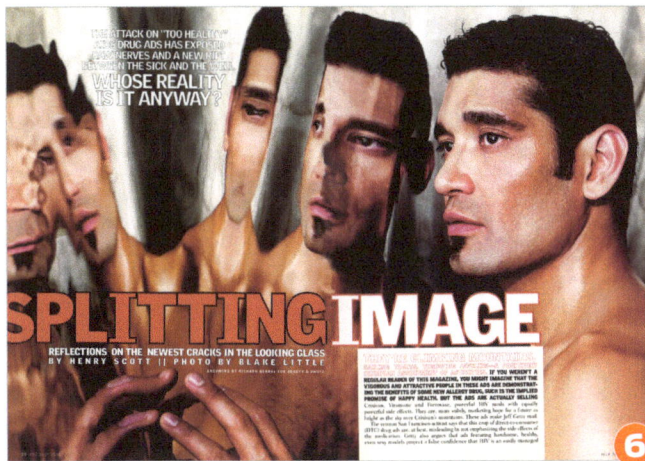

SPLITTING IMAGE

REFLECTIONS ON THE NEWEST CRACKS IN THE LOOKING GLASS
BY HENRY SCOTT || PHOTO BY BLAKE LITTLE

(6)

July

COVER: Are the models in HIV drug ads too healthy-looking? Some activists are pushing to ban the glamorous face of AIDS many advertisers are selling (**6**). **INSIDE:** The winners of POZ's Rage and Remembrance Literary Contest; what undetectable really means. **PLUS:** MTV commercials parody public service ads about sexually transmitted infections.

September

COVER: POZ presents The Death Issue. **INSIDE:** A lesson from Keith Haring on the art of dying; eight artists and activists on making death work for you; assisted suicide makes a controversial comeback (**8**). **PLUS:** AIDS photography's greatest hits.

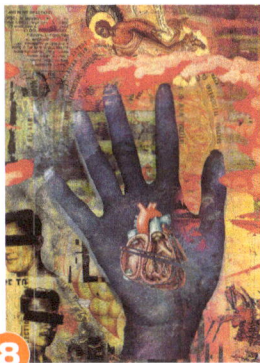

(8)

November

COVER: Even as they debunk a much-hyped case of superinfection, researchers have finally launched a study to prove whether people with HIV can be "twice bitten" by

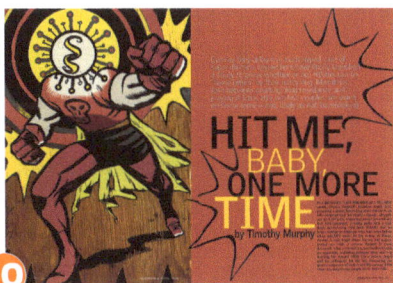

HIT ME, BABY ONE MORE TIME by Timothy Murphy

(10)

the virus (**10**). **INSIDE:** How St. Vincent's Hospital in New York City's Greenwich Village came to the rescue of people with HIV during the darkest days of AIDS as well as survivors of the 9/11 terrorist attack. **PLUS:** Congress takes on a queer barebacker.

August

COVER: Mike Barr's special report on structured treatment interruptions. **INSIDE:** Chicago-based Dance for Life helps dancers with pricey prescriptions and doctor's visits; punk rocker–turned-writer Joe Westmoreland talks his debut novel, *Tramps Like Us*, and living with HIV (**7**); a therapist on why HIV isn't always to blame when it comes to not finding love. **PLUS:** POZ recaps 20 years of the AIDS epidemic.

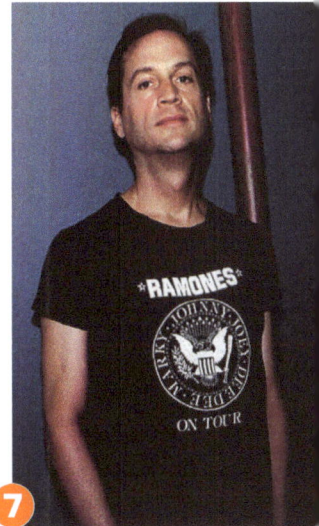

(7)

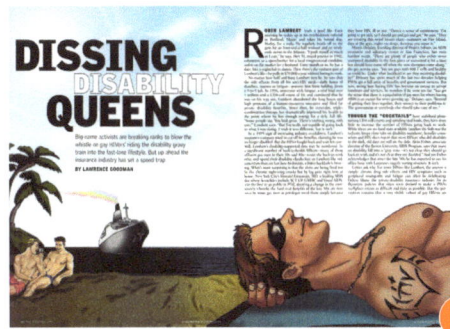

DISSING DISABILITY QUEENS

BY LAWRENCE GODWIN

(9)

October

COVER: Five women activists question the prevalence of girl-to-guy transmission of HIV. **INSIDE:** Some activists want to blow the whistle on healthy people with HIV living large off disability benefits (**9**); why are people with HIV getting shingles? **PLUS:** Controversial Senator Jesse Helms retires.

December

COVER: The most memorable AIDS moments from 2001. **INSIDE:** A lab that's rebuilding immune systems may help turn ordinary people with HIV into long-term nonprogressors; China breaks its long silence on its exploding AIDS epidemic, but is it too late for PWAs? **PLUS:** David Welch has a new heart and is blazing a trail for transplants for people with HIV (**11**).

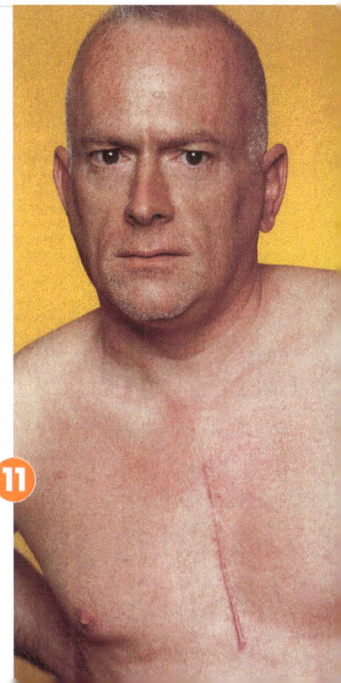

(11)

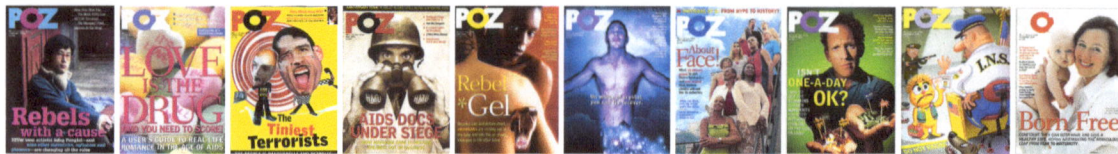

2002

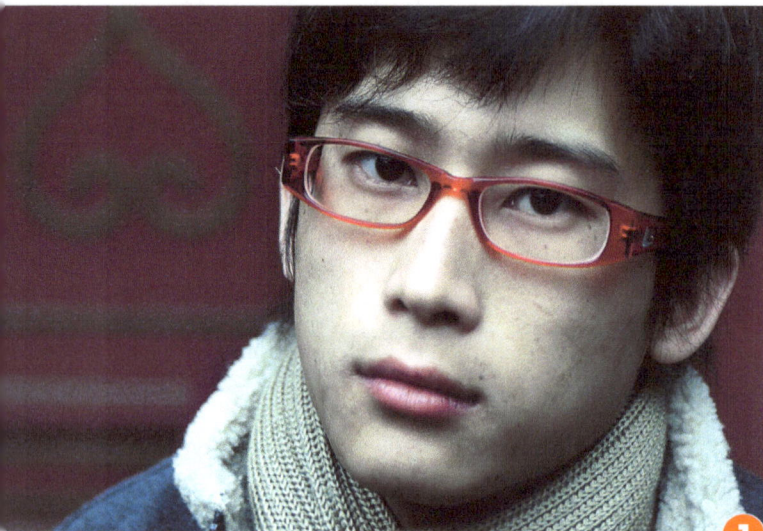

January

COVER: Song Pengfei is a speaker, writer and activist who is living with HIV in Beijing. He and nine other mavericks, agitators and pioneers are changing the rules for treatment, prevention and activism (**1**). **INSIDE:** The feds block imports of an injectable gel used to reverse facial wasting due to meds; Paul Harris runs a mile with the Olympic torch. **PLUS:** Treatment trials and tribulations in Uganda.

February/March

COVER: A user's guide to real-life romance in the age of AIDS (**2**). **INSIDE:** Sky-high prices, exploding enrollment and new national priorities are bankrupting ADAP; Catholics for condoms. **PLUS:** The announcement of the first-ever series of successful liver transplants in five people living with HIV and coinfected with hep B, C or both.

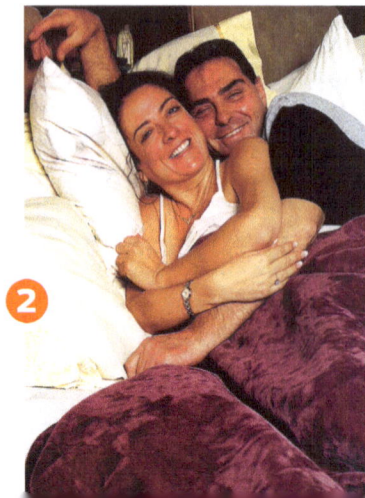

April

COVER: *The People v. David Pasquarelli and Michael Petrelis.* **INSIDE:** President Bush has stacked his AIDS council with anti-condom crusaders (**3**); why needle exchange is failing in Vancouver. **PLUS:** The SMART trial will monitor 6,000 people living with HIV for an average of seven years to determine the long-term effects of treatment interruptions.

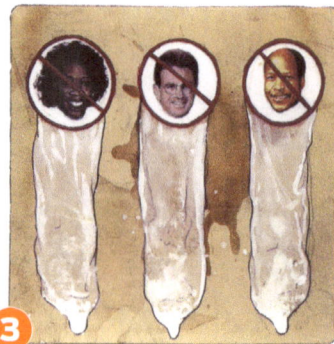

May

COVER: How managed care is driving the best AIDS doctors out of the business (**4**). **INSIDE:** Divinely driven Dick Scanlan brings *Thoroughly Modern Millie* to Broadway; forget your fears and make your mouth happy with good oral health. **PLUS:** How to get a grip on HIV intimacy issues.

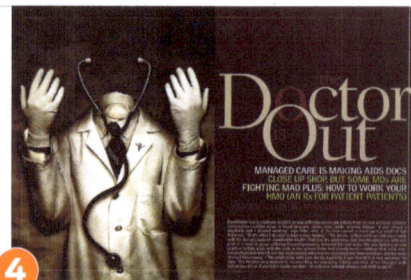

June

COVER: Microbicides may soon make their way out of the (test) tube and into the sheets. **INSIDE:** How to spell relief for HIV-related pain; tips for getting your man to go downtown. **PLUS:** Top AIDS researchers tell all from the 14th International AIDS Conference in Barcelona (**5**).

July/August

COVER: How crystal meth's primal allure speeds transmission and resistance. **INSIDE:** Viral resistance is a fact of life, but it's no reason to flush your HIV meds down the toilet (6); a college freshman faces up to 45 years for not disclosing before sex. **PLUS:** A collection of photos from Camp Heartland reveals spirited campers in a safe space.

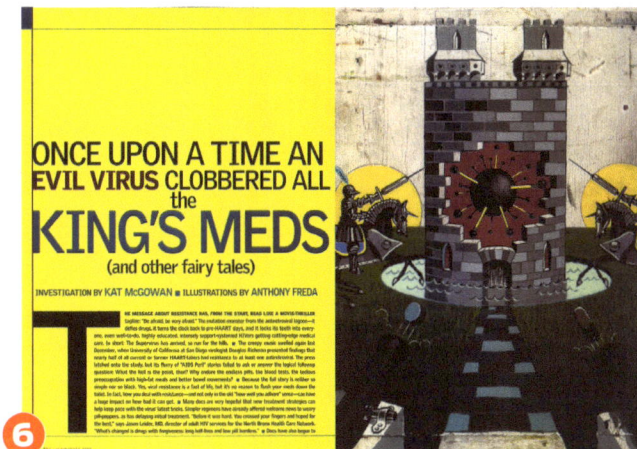

September

COVER: Meet 10 New Yorkers who've taken a good, hard look at themselves—and find a beauty inside that HIV can't take away. **INSIDE:** Should courts force parents to put their kids on HIV medications?; our anonymous columnist wonders whether lipodystrophy will give her away (7). **PLUS:** The problem with protease inhibitors.

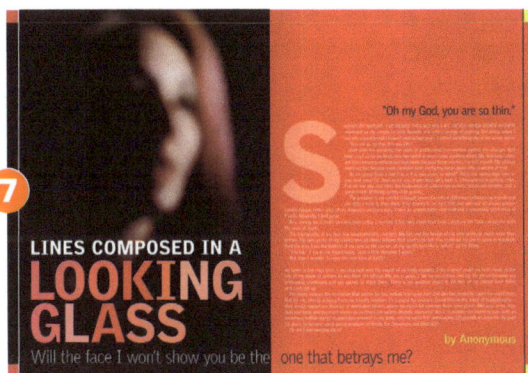

October

COVER: Mark Leydorf is on a quest to get all the vitamins and other nutrients he needs with as few pills as possible (8). **INSIDE:** People living with HIV in rural America have to make like pioneers to get the care and support they need; an ex–porn star's second act leads to health and happiness. **PLUS:** Sean Strub on sexual abuse, HIV and why the Catholic priest scandal hit home.

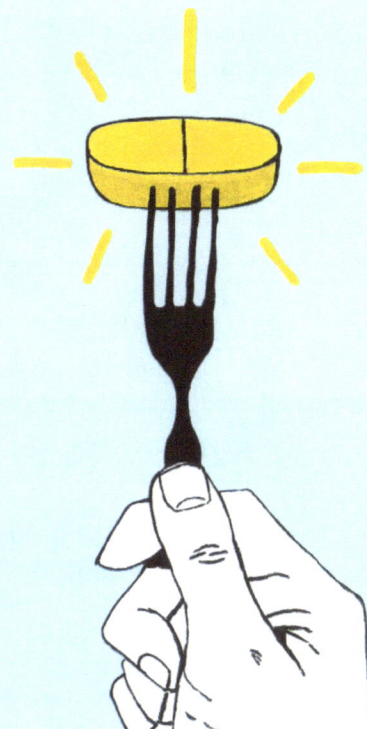

November

COVER: Kami is a muppet with HIV on South Africa's *Sesame Street* who teaches acceptance and love. So why are Republican congressmen trying to stop her from coming to America (9)? **INSIDE:** Meet the folks advising George W. Bush on how to stop HIV—and doing everything they can to roll back 20 years of condom sense. **PLUS:** A kitty-killing HIV study starts an animal-rights catfight.

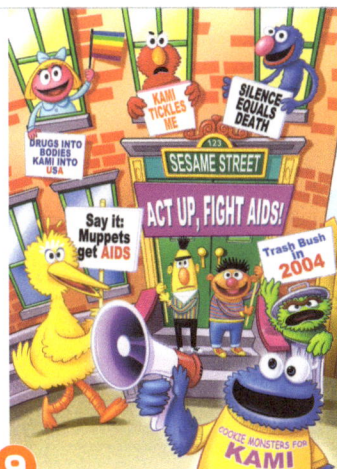

December

COVER: Dawn Averitt and other women living with HIV are making the miraculous leap from fear to maternity. **INSIDE:** Visual AIDS, the group that gave us Day With(out) Art and the Red Ribbon, returns to its (grass) roots (10). **PLUS:** Kansas City star Jane Fowler lights 67 birthday candles and a flame under her fellow seniors with HIV.

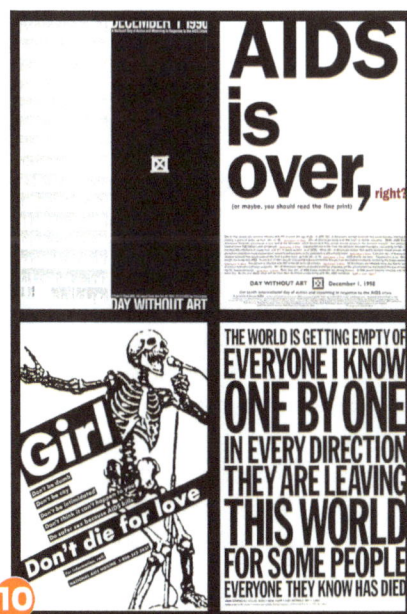

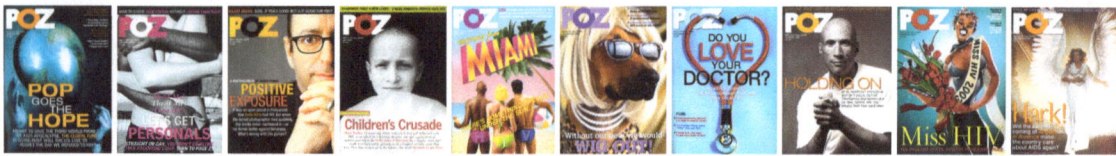

2003

January

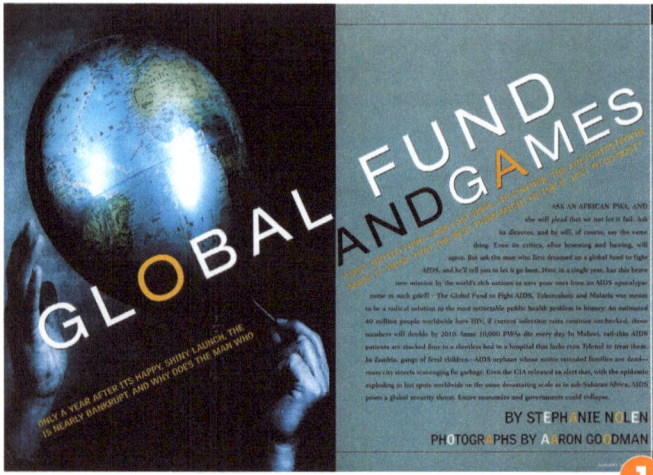

COVER: High hopes that the Global Fund could head off a worldwide AIDS catastrophe are being dashed as rich nations fall short of their promises and poor ones falter on accountability (1). **INSIDE:** For those with hepatitis C, once-a-week pegylated interferon treatment is an improvement over thrice-weekly shots of alpha interferon. **PLUS:** An update on founder Sean Strub's health.

February/March

COVER: POZ serves up a feast of 53 hot personals in time for Valentine's Day. **INSIDE:** The 20-minute HIV test is here; why Michael Musto thinks *The Hours* may be the best AIDS movie ever; five ways to keep down the cost of your co-pays (2). **PLUS:** Athletes with HIV remind the Gay Games of their positive founder's golden vision.

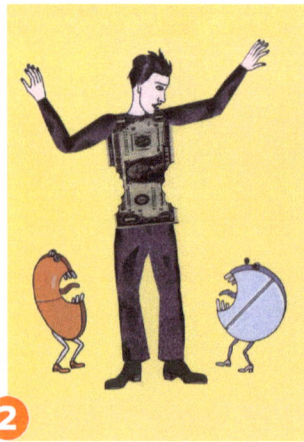

April

COVER: When photographer Herb Ritts died suddenly in December, the media never mentioned AIDS, let alone his battle against blindness (3). **INSIDE:** A new law in California requires HMOs to refer people living with HIV to an HIV specialist; a passionate practice-what-you-preach pastor gets tested for HIV in front of his congregation. **PLUS:** How to lose your job without losing your insurance.

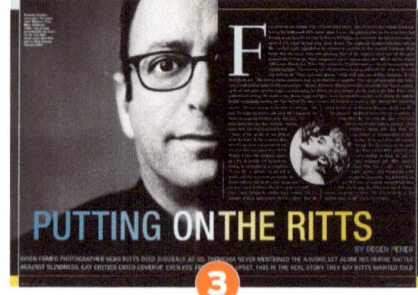

May

COVER: A photo essay captures "Romania's AIDS orphans" who survived genocide in 1991 and now need life-saving meds. **INSIDE:** Miss America 1998 talks condom sense to Miss America 2003 (4); people with HIV seeking a liver transplant face a long wait and the world's highest-stakes waiting list. **PLUS:** How did a nice Iowa grandma living with HIV end up in an Indonesian jail?

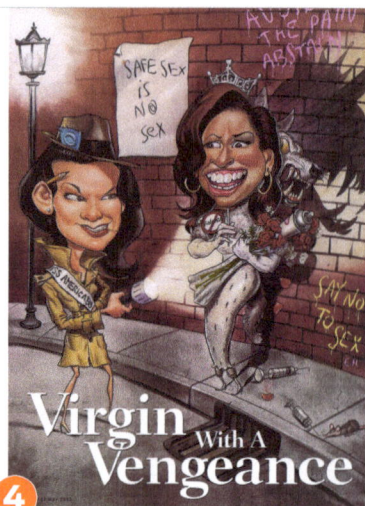

June

COVER: Minorities are competing with one another for funding to fight the nation's highest AIDS rate in Miami (5). **INSIDE:** A sexual misconduct scandal threatens the career of Scott Hitt, the prominent AIDS doctor who heads the American Academy of HIV Medicine. **PLUS:** Filmmaker Rory Kennedy (RFK's youngest) brings global AIDS to HBO with the documentary *Pandemic: Facing AIDS*.

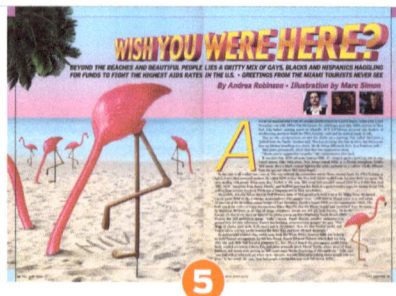

July/August

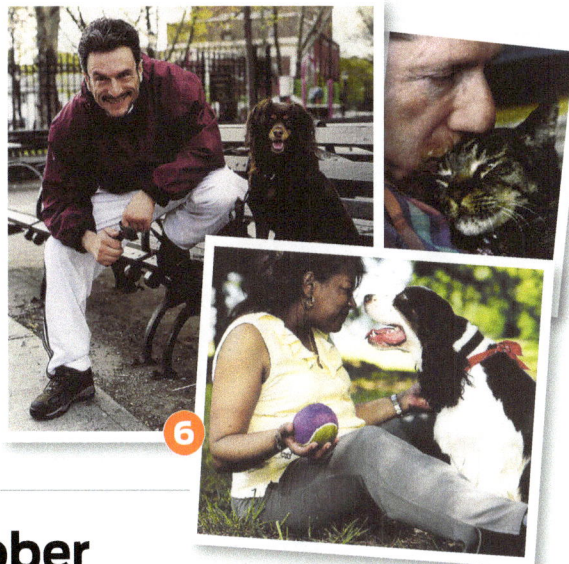

COVER: A tribute to our pets, who comfort us when we're sick and play with us when we're well (**6**). **INSIDE:** A hormone replacement therapy scare leaves women with HIV wondering how to manage menopause; the rhythms of late musician and activist Fela Anikulapo-Kuti, who died of AIDS-related illness, go on. **PLUS:** A once-a-day-pill called pre-exposure prophylaxis (PrEP) could help prevent HIV transmission.

September

COVER: POZ explores the relationship between doctors and their patients. **INSIDE:** Hilary Beard tries to figure out why HIV is disproportionately affecting Black teenage girls (**7**); a last-ditch plan to save the Global AIDS Fund. **PLUS:** How to read drug resistance tests.

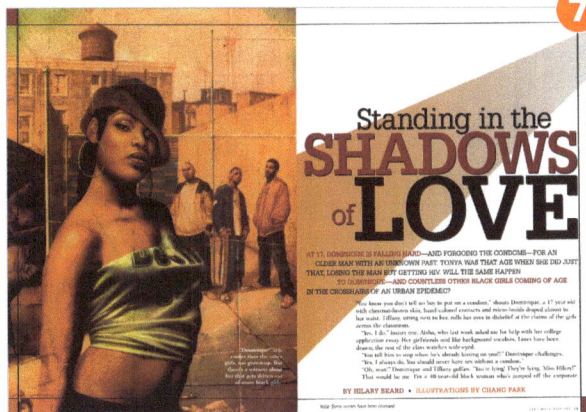

October

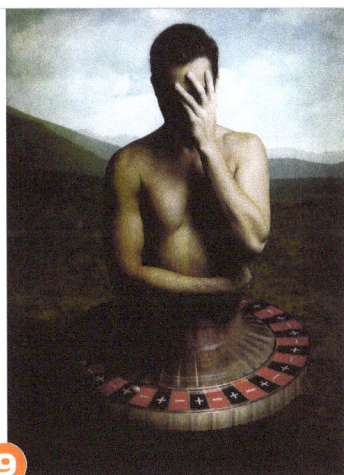

COVER: Out of treatment options, Norfleet Person desperately waits for the arrival of salvage therapy (**8**). **INSIDE:** What happens to people with HIV in Baghdad now that Iraq's single public AIDS facility has been destroyed? **PLUS:** Columnist Nurse Know-It-All serves up some cold advice regarding antiretroviral treatment and her two favorite vices, booze and tobacco.

November

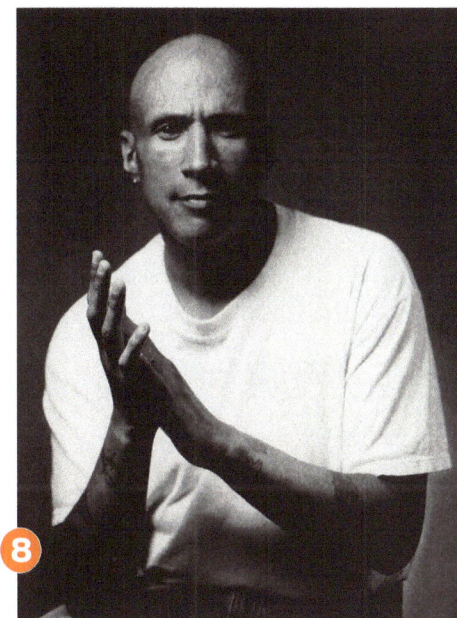

COVER: Miss HIV Stigma-Free is crowned in Botswana. **INSIDE:** New York City neighborhoods Harlem and Chelsea are worlds apart when it comes to the rate of AIDS-related deaths; why did so many HIV-negative gay men seroconvert after testing VaxGen's failed vaccine despite safe-sex counseling and support (**9**)? **PLUS:** Treatment news from the International AIDS Society confab in Paris.

December

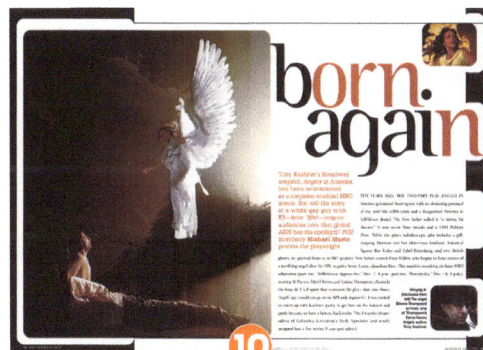

COVER: Columnist Michael Musto catches up with playwright Tony Kushner on the movie adaptation of *Angels in America* (**10**). **INSIDE:** Five Los Angelenos on living with HIV and beating addiction; a peewee football coach loses his job to HIV stigma, but the team's parents get him back in the game. **PLUS:** Tips on how to read and understand HIV research.

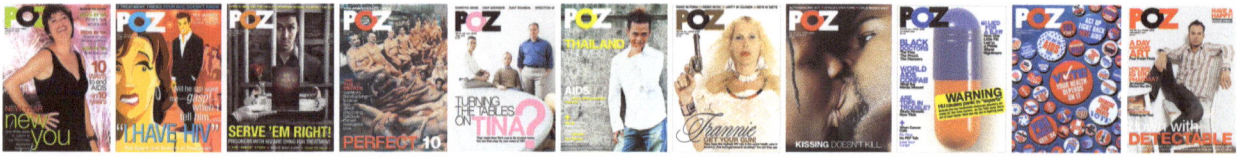

2004

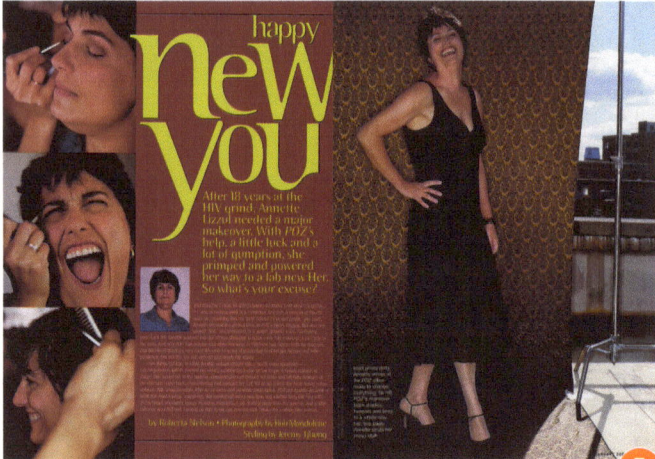

January

COVER: Longtime survivor Annette Lizzul gets a POZ makeover (**1**). **INSIDE:** The CDC's "prevention for positives" campaign is shaming gay men with HIV; 10 ways to end AIDS in 10 years. **PLUS:** HIV-positive Richard Brodsky runs the New York City marathon after being diagnosed with cancer.

February/March

COVER: Just in time for Valentine's Day, our sex guru gets people with HIV to spill their disclosure tips. **INSIDE:** Three treatment tricks that may go against your doctor's orders (**2**); POZ founder Sean Strub shares how he climbed out of depression. **PLUS:** Spill your bedroom secrets in POZ's first-ever sex survey.

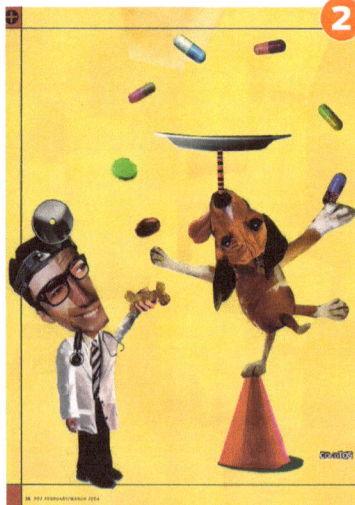

April

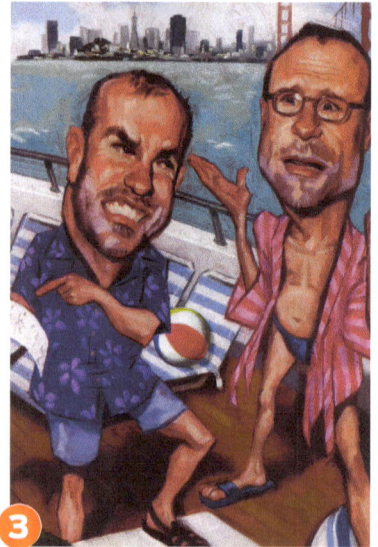

COVER: Our survival guide for inmates with HIV. **INSIDE:** What happens when holistic healers must choose between getting sick and taking the cocktail; how lies and HIV turned an internet hookup into a major courtroom drama (**3**). **PLUS:** *Queer as Folk*'s writers talk about HIV's role in season 4.

May

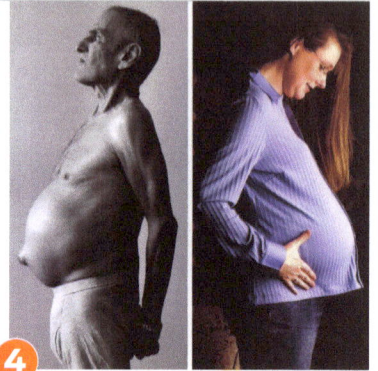

COVER: Our 10th anniversary cover installation with artist Spencer Tunick features 80 people living with HIV—baring it all! **INSIDE:** A year-by-year chronicle of the past 10 years of POZ; catching up with people who have appeared on the cover of POZ. **PLUS:** Larry Kramer and Dawn Averitt remind us of the gift of life (**4**).

June

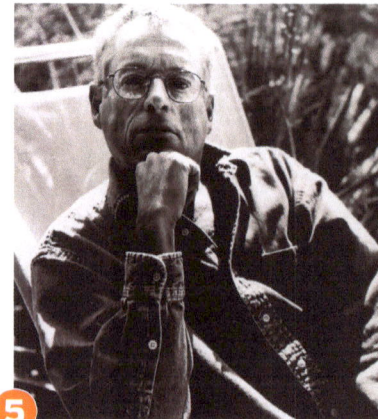

COVER: Activists get New York City to face its growing crystal meth problem. **INSIDE:** At AIDSWatch, advocates went to the Capitol to demand federal dollars for treatment; the link between HIV and domestic abuse and how to get help. **PLUS:** AIDS Memorial Quilt founder Cleve Jones is fired from the organization that manages the 40,000-plus hand-stitched panels (**5**).

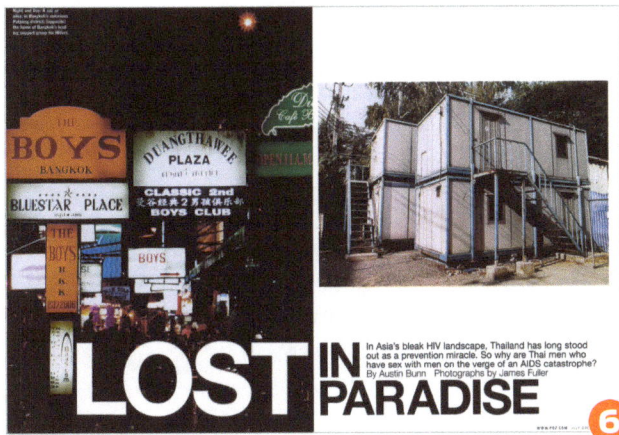

July

COVER: Men who have sex with men in Thailand are on the verge of an AIDS catastrophe (**6**). **INSIDE:** Residents of Broadway House in Newark produce their first-ever art show; can you forgive the person who gave you HIV? **PLUS:** Read the results of our debut sex survey.

August

COVER: Trans people have the highest rates of HIV and the worst health care—learn how they're fighting back (**7**). **INSIDE:** How open dialogue about HIV in Uganda led to plummeting HIV rates; New York's Public Theater revives Larry Kramer's *The Normal Heart*. **PLUS:** A blow-by-blow from the front lines of the biggest AIDS demo in Washington, DC, in a decade.

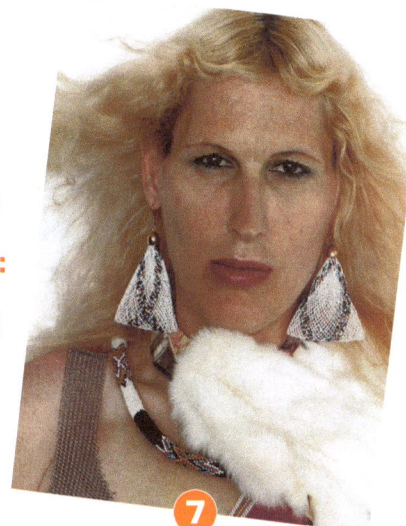

September

COVER: Exploring the phenomenon known as "the down low." **INSIDE:** The AIDS Treatment Coalition is making pharma and the feds listen to your treatment needs; a step-by-step guide on how a pill gets to market (**8**). **PLUS:** By cuddling kiddies, Alicia Keys, Oprah and other celebs are putting a human face on AIDS in Africa.

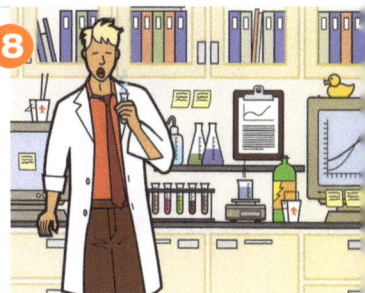

October

COVER: How—and why—the federal government and top docs have shelved a potentially lifesaving HIV medication called hydroxyurea. **INSIDE:** An HIV-positive man's terrifying trials after telling his trick he's HIV negative; six nights in Bangkok at the 15th International AIDS Conference. **PLUS:** The nation's top Black AIDS doctors are uniting to tailor research and treatment to African Americans (**9**).

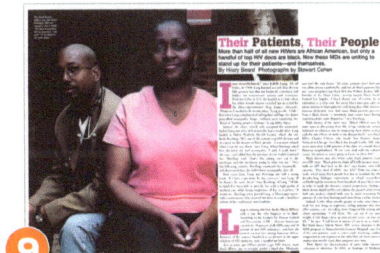

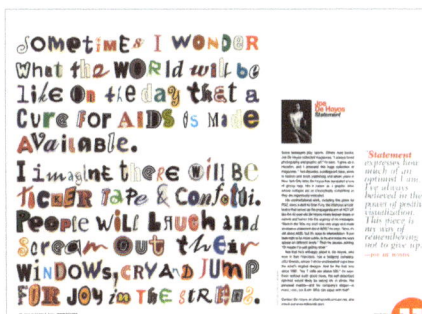

December

COVER: Aiming to escape side effects and preserve future options, more and more people living with HIV are daring to live with a detectable virus. **INSIDE:** To commemorate Day With(out) Art, four HIV-positive artists share work about life and love with HIV (**11**); a new exposé on the greed and corruption of big pharma. **PLUS:** What it's like to climb Mt. Kilimanjaro while living with HIV.

November

COVER: POZ's special report on the 2004 election breaks down the issues (**10**). **INSIDE:** Shari Margolese's son busts her for taking her "herbal" meds; Florida has a new snare tactic for sex workers living with HIV. **PLUS:** The scoop on entry inhibitors—the next big class of HIV drugs.

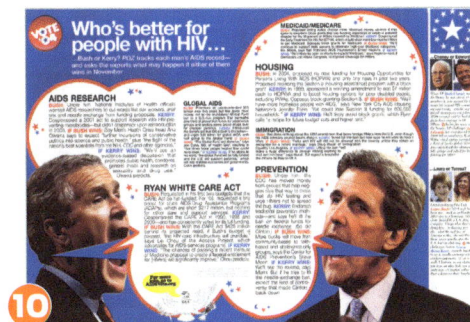

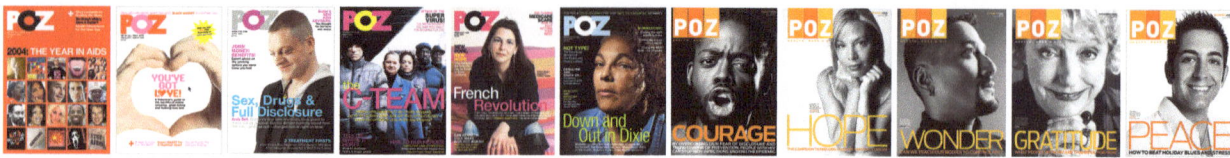

The top row shows POZ magazine covers.

THE YEAR IN POZ

2005

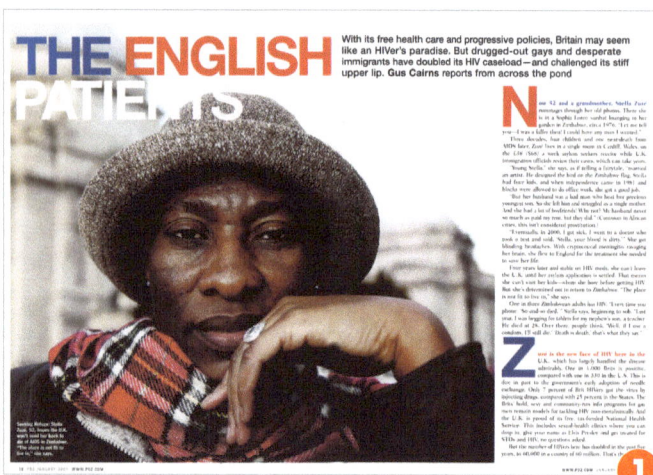

THE ENGLISH PATIENTS

With its free health care and progressive policies, Britain may seem like an HIVer's paradise. But drugged-out gays and desperate immigrants have doubled its HIV caseload—and challenged its stiff upper lip. Gus Cairns reports from across the pond.

1

January

COVER: The top HIV/AIDS-related stories of 2004. **INSIDE:** A report on the HIV epidemic across the pond in Britain (**1**); Greg Louganis on dealing with depression and the healing power of his dogs; six superheroes of 2004. **PLUS:** Shawn Decker and Gwenn Barringer's wedding.

February/March

COVER: A Valentine's Day guide to finding romance online and making love last (**2**). **INSIDE:** HIV meds on the black market; 20 foods that boost immune energy; butt pad underwear to boost the booty. **PLUS:** Brent Mower discloses his status and climbs the Great Wall of China to raise money for amfAR's TREAT Asia program.

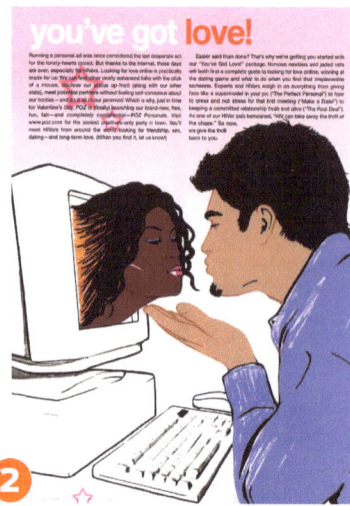

you've got love!

2

April

COVER: After announcing publicly that he is living with HIV, Erasure front man Andy Bell talks to POZ about blow, blow jobs and barebacking (**3**). **INSIDE:** Expert advice on how to find work, get health care coverage and keep your disability benefits; there's new hope for a therapeutic vaccine. **PLUS:** The first one-pill, once-a-day HIV treatment is in the works.

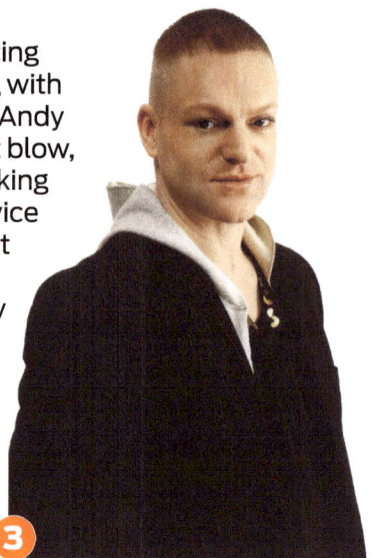

3

May

COVER: Jules Levin leads the fight for those with HIV and hep C coinfection. **INSIDE:** A tribute to Sylvester, the disco diva who braved '80s stigma to sound the alarm about the epidemic (**4**); a profile of activist Esther Boucicault, who in 1999 became the first woman living with HIV in Haiti to publicly announce her status. **PLUS:** A breakdown of the media sensationalism over the latest supervirus story.

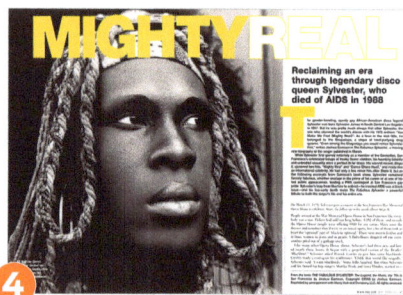

MIGHTY REAL

Reclaiming an era through legendary disco queen Sylvester, who died of AIDS in 1988

4

June

COVER: A controversial group of French women living with HIV believe that transmitting HIV is a crime and turn to right-wing politicians for justice. **INSIDE:** Michael Musto interviews fashion designer Kenneth Cole and Mathilde Krim, MD, as Cole steps into Krim's shoes as the new chairman of the board of amfAR (**5**). **PLUS:** How to get the most out of your interaction with the receptionist at your doctor's office.

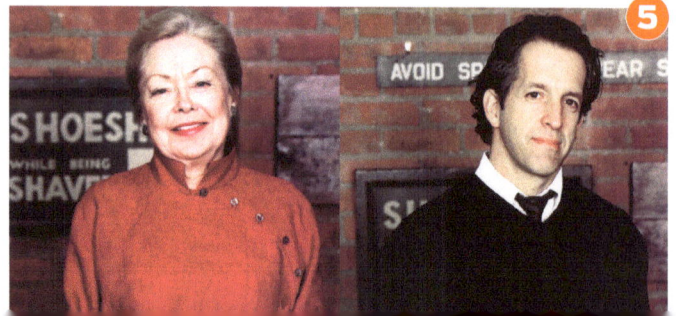

5

July

COVER: Michelle Lampkin weighs in on the difficulties of living with HIV in the South (6). **INSIDE:** The winners of the POZ fiction and poetry contest; 20 years of the AIDS Walk; legal expert Catherine Hanssens on the medical rights of inmates. **PLUS:** Grammy-nominated jazz pianist Fred Hersch shares his tips for carrying his HIV meds on the road.

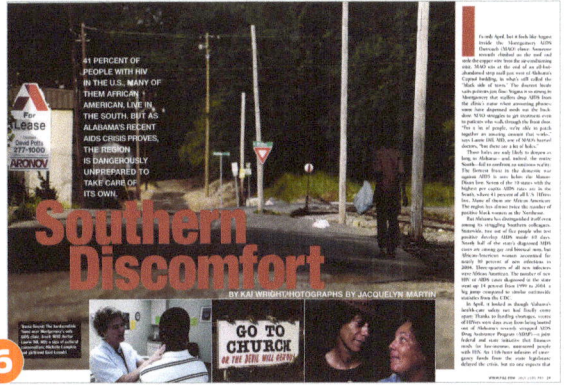

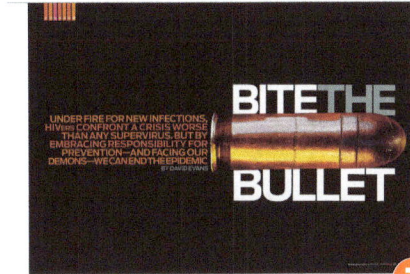

Southern Discomfort
BY KAI WRIGHT/PHOTOGRAPHS BY JACQUELYN MARTIN

August

COVER: Kwame "Blackkat" Banks, the first African American to win American Leatherman. **INSIDE:** Focusing on viral hot spots and launching reality-based interventions to end the epidemic (7); Spencer Cox writes about getting over the AIDS crisis. **PLUS:** Mastering meditation can empower your immune system.

September

COVER: Dawnmarie Sims shares what HIV has taught her about hope. **INSIDE:** Catching up with Raven Lopez, who appeared on our August/September 1996 cover; Charles King reveals his vision for the Campaign to End AIDS (C2EA), a cross-country caravan of HIV advocates heading to Washington, DC, for five days of action (8). **PLUS:** Meet 10 people living with HIV who are part of the C2EA caravan (9).

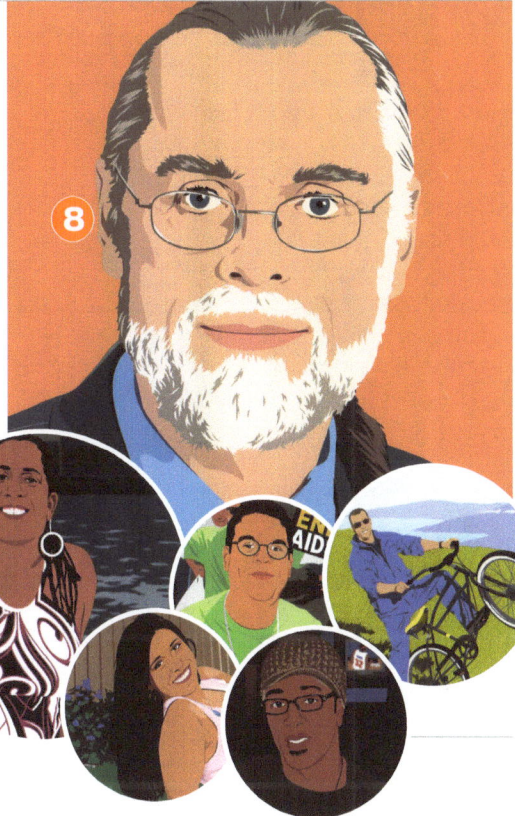

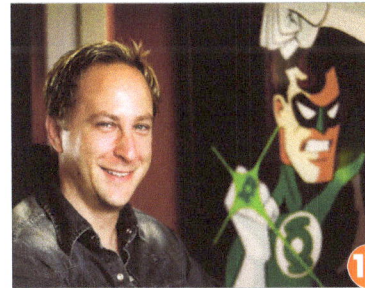

October

COVER: Gerard Thai on the wonder of HIV. **INSIDE:** A look at the future of immune-based therapies; River Huston wonders whether disclosing her status will hurt her sex-toy business. **PLUS:** Comic-book creator Darren Davis on Zak Raven, the studly, HIV-positive hero of his next comic, *Lost Raven* (10).

November

COVER: Jane Fowler is a 70-year-old HIV-positive grandmother who can't stop talking about sex (11). **INSIDE:** POZ sets the table for a Thanksgiving feast and a discussion about gratitude and HIV; five tips for disclosure. **PLUS:** Charting the odds of transmission during mixed-status sex without a condom.

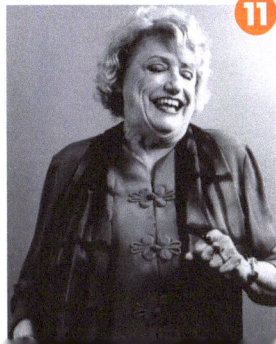

December

COVER: Juliano Innocenti finds peace with his HIV. **INSIDE:** How to beat the seasonal blues—especially around the holidays; the HIV community reacts to Hurricane Katrina (12); POZ remembers editor and columnist LeRoy Whitfield. **PLUS:** Five great treatment developments of 2005.

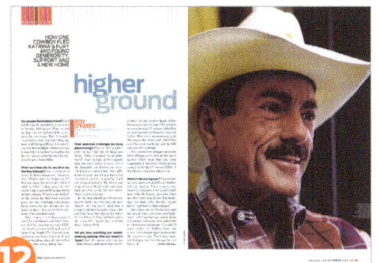

higher ground

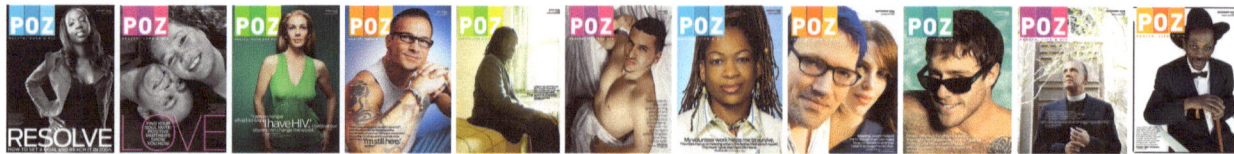

2006

January

COVER: Activist Marvelyn Brown shares her New Year's resolution. **INSIDE:** Strategies for making bold resolutions that will last all year long; Edwin Cameron, South Africa's first openly HIV-positive high-court judge, issues a verdict on his country's HIV epidemic (**1**). **PLUS:** How safe is oral sex?

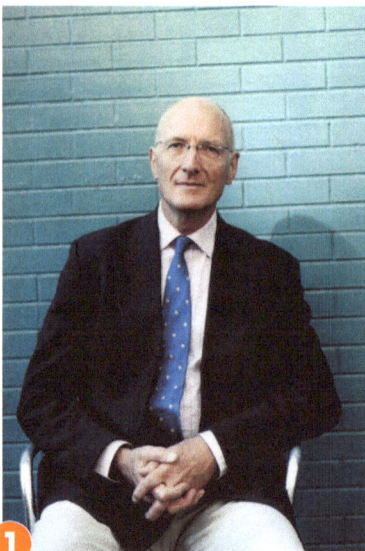

February/March

WHETHER POPPING THEIR MEDS OR POPPING THE QUESTION, THESE COUPLES FOUND LOVE AMID HIV. REBECCA MINNICH ASKS THEM—AND A BUNCH OF THERAPISTS AND COUNSELORS—HOW YOU CAN DO IT, TOO

a positive attraction

COVER: Millie Malave and Bryan Fleury, both living with HIV, discuss how they found romance despite self-doubt (**2**). **INSIDE:** Ten Black AIDS warriors to watch; how to navigate Medicare's new prescription drug maze. **PLUS:** Figure skater Rudy Galindo dishes about how he discloses his status.

April

COVER: POZ names its "Anonymous" columnist, Regan Hofmann, as editor-in-chief of the magazine. **INSIDE:** Crime novelist John Morgan Wilson reveals his own HIV story line; why does denialism—asserting that HIV does not cause AIDS—continue to have appeal (**3**)? **PLUS:** The double whammy of herpes and HIV.

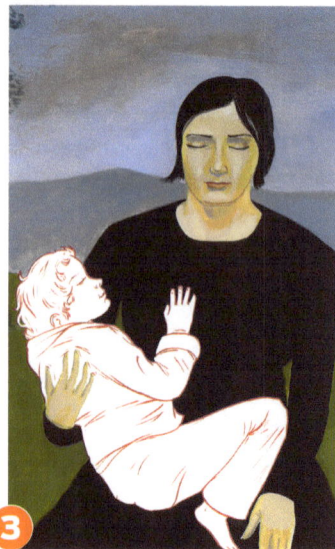

May

medicine men

COVER: Bob Bowers, the president of HIVictorious Inc., shares what it's like to be a long-term survivor. **INSIDE:** Peter Staley and Tim Horn—the dynamic duo behind AIDSmeds.com—discuss the science and activism behind HIV treatment (**4**); Bono sees (RED) with his new AIDS-fundraising brand. **PLUS:** Why did AIDS never star on *Will & Grace*?

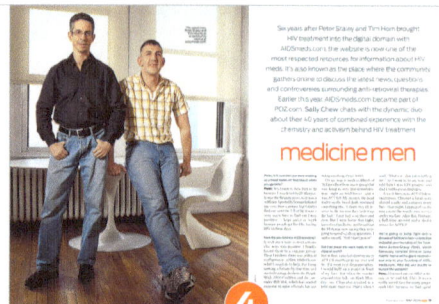

June

COVER: Catching up with jazz singer Andy Bey, who returned to music after his HIV diagnosis in 1994 (**5**). **INSIDE:** After 25 years of the AIDS epidemic, our temptation to view the virus as largely a foreign policy issue is a deadly domestic mistake; New York City's bold new HIV testing initiative. **PLUS:** Should you disclose at the workplace?

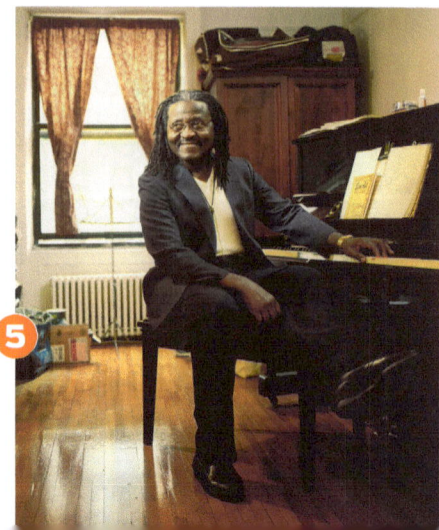

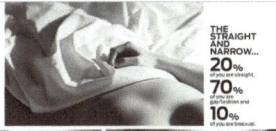

SPEAKING OF SEX…

POZ asked you, our HIV positive readers, how having HIV has affected your sex lives—delving into topics from disclosure to safer sex. Nearly a thousand of you (85% men, 14% women and 1% transgendered people) responded, revealing the innermost secrets of your behavior in the boudoir. Wonder how you measure up? Read on…

THE STRAIGHT AND NARROW…
20% of you are straight.
70% of you are straight.
10% of you are gay, lesbian or bisexual.

68 PERCENT of you are single. If you're in the market, try checking out POZ Personals on POZ.com.

THE TIES THAT BIND

July

COVER: Todd Murray on why he started Hope's Voice, a national nonprofit that serves youth living with HIV. **INSIDE:** Prosecuting people living with HIV who don't disclose their status before sex; POZ readers share the secrets of their sex lives (**6**). **PLUS:** Finding the perfect support group.

August

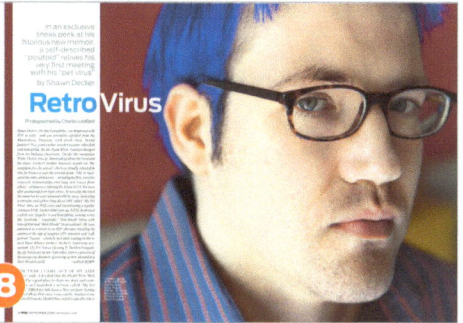

COVER: Activist, HIV educator and mom Nicole Guide and 17 other HIV survival experts share secrets to prevailing with HIV despite dangerous environments and significant odds (**7**). **INSIDE:** After losing three sons to AIDS, Martha MacGuffie, MD, fights back; HIV and the Boy Scouts. **PLUS:** The San Francisco Department of Health launches the nation's first text-message prevention campaign.

September

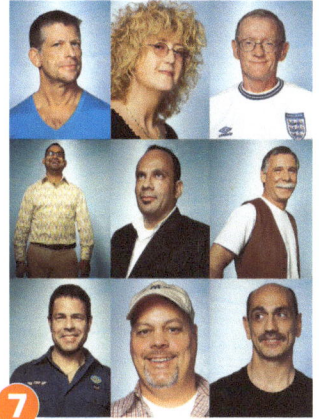

COVER: Serodiscordant couple and HIV educators Shawn Decker and Gwenn Barringer. **INSIDE:** An excerpt from Decker's new memoir, *My Pet Virus* (**8**); POZ offers a guide to solvency to help with the high medical cost of living with HIV and past financial mistakes. **PLUS:** Take our survey about AIDS activism.

October

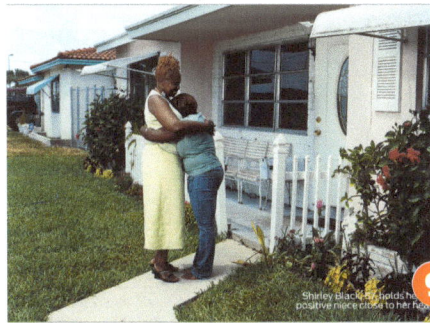

Shirley Black-Brown holds her positive niece close to her face.

COVER: Born with HIV, Jake Glaser talks about living with the virus and the death of his mom, the founder of the Elizabeth Glaser Pediatric AIDS Foundation. **INSIDE:** In families living with HIV, older relatives learn to be parents again (**9**). **PLUS:** How the Bill Gates and Warren Buffet AIDS money will trickle down—or not.

November

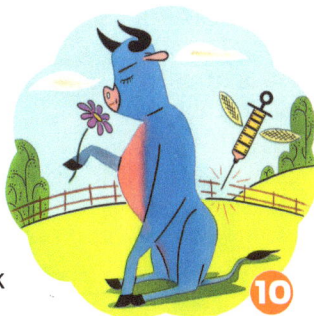

COVER: The Reverend Dr. Keith Riddle explains how contracting HIV actually strengthened his faith. **INSIDE:** Kay Warren, wife of the pastor and founder of Saddleback Church, teaches spiritual leaders worldwide to rethink their position on AIDS; keeping your cool while keeping your hormone levels up (**10**). **PLUS:** Housewives of Brazil become unlikely safe-sex educators.

December

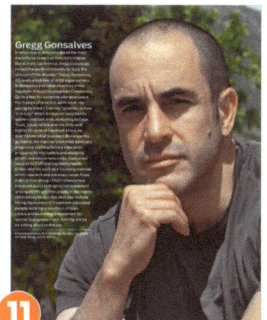

Gregg Gonsalves

COVER: William "Billy" Dickerson, a resident of the HIV care facility Rivington House in New York City, shares why he wears a suit every day. **INSIDE:** 35 Ones to Watch: From Malawi to Mississippi, these folks are helping put an end to AIDS (**11**); new HIV drugs mean some long-term survivors can become undetectable. **PLUS:** Despite HIV's "manageability," treatment still comes with numerous side effects.

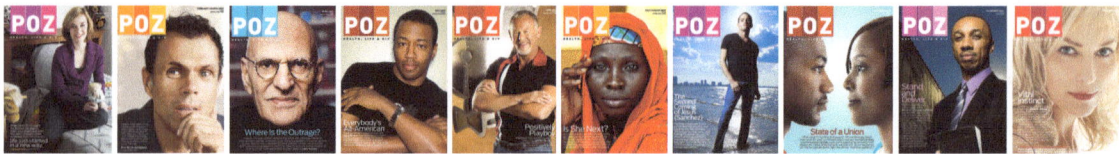

THE YEAR IN POZ

2007

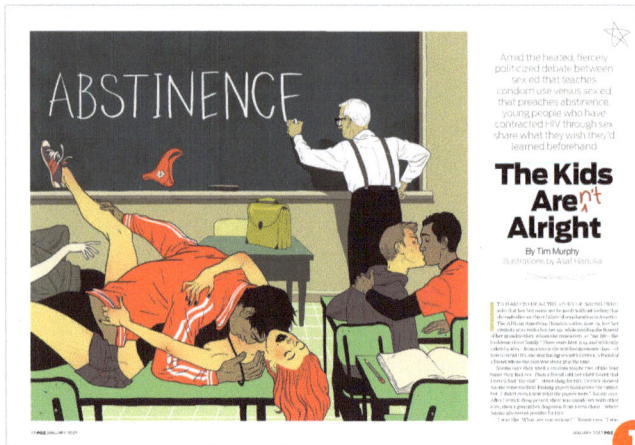

January

COVER: Chelsea Gulden fights to protect her HIV-negative child from the stigma many HIV-positive parents face. **INSIDE:** For at-risk kids, the real AIDS crisis is the lack of sex education (**1**); the CDC wants to normalize HIV testing. **PLUS:** A schoolteacher living with HIV in Alabama instructs his students in safer sex 101 after grading their math homework.

February/March

COVER: On A&E's *Designing Blind*, Eric Brun-Sanglard is an A-list interior designer living with HIV who lost his sight 11 years ago (**2**). **INSIDE:** Move to the healing power of house music; will gender-changing hormones interact with your HIV regimen? **PLUS:** A look at serosorting—the tactic of exclusively selecting sexual partners of the same HIV status.

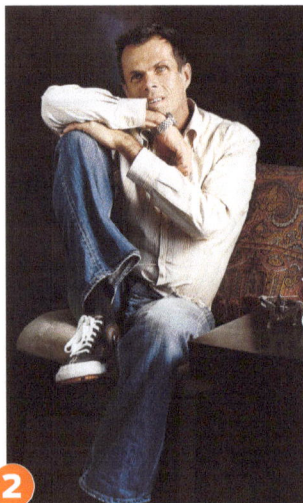

April

COVER: Larry Kramer gives a rebel-rousing speech, but is the world ready to listen again (**3**)? **INSIDE:** People over 50 account for at least 10% of new infections; hairdressers in Memphis trim away HIV-related stigma. **PLUS:** ACT UP New York turns 20.

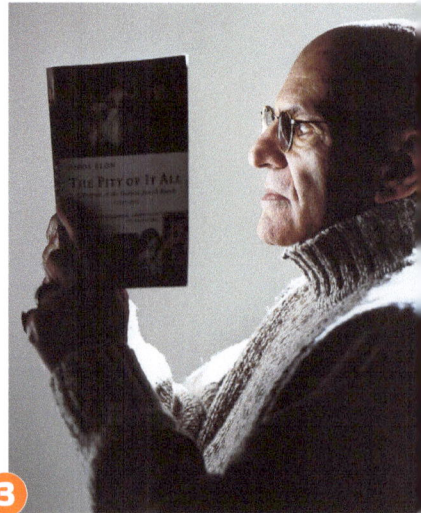

May

COVER: Larry Bryant is a former all-American football star living with HIV who has been drafted to a new team looking to end AIDS (**4**). **INSIDE:** physically challenged people living with HIV share how they've disabled stigma and self-doubt; Puerto Rico faces AIDS funding corruption and a health care catastrophe. **PLUS:** Meet several undocumented immigrants living with HIV who are struggling to live stateside.

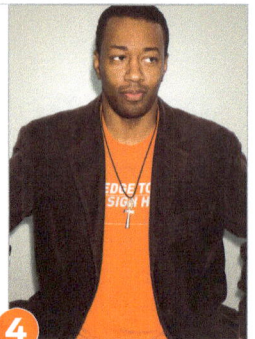

June

COVER: VP of Playboy Entertainment Jeffrey Jenest—who is openly gay and living with HIV—gets his own centerfold and talks about the often condomless world of adult entertainment and his own journey with the virus (**5**). **INSIDE:** Jenna Bush's new book about AIDS sounds suspiciously like her dad's old policies; for this brave breed of mountaineers living with HIV, the only way is up. **PLUS:** Why it's been so difficult to conduct the necessary studies to prove—or disprove—the benefits of pre-exposure prophylaxis, or PrEP.

July/August

COVER: The rampant spread of HIV through sexual violence and rape is an overlooked war crime of the civil conflict in the Democratic Republic of Congo (**6**). **INSIDE:** Purveyors of alleged HIV treatments have built a lucrative market in India, where stigma and poverty keep millions from proper care; a Ryan White CARE Act scorecard. **PLUS:** Product (RED) wants you to shop till AIDS drops—but critics aren't buying it.

September

COVER: Aspiring TV anchor Jesus "Jesse" Sanchez recasts his HIV diagnosis into a fierce new ambition. **INSIDE:** Sexual and religious repression in the Caribbean have spawned deadly homophobia and fueled HIV transmission; bone-building tips and tricks; kids at risk for HIV bend it like Beckham in South Africa. **PLUS:** Disclosing her HIV status boosted Lora Tucker's health and improved her life (**7**).

October

COVER: As the African-American community rallies to fight its exploding HIV rate, straight Black women (like Fortunata Kasege) and gay Black men (like Kali Lindsey) are uniting to fight AIDS (**8**). **INSIDE:** The career of self-proclaimed AIDS diva Sheryl Lee Ralph; how to launch a support network. **PLUS:** Beating HIV drug resistance to the punch.

November

COVER: The Reverend Stacey Latimer is throwing the good book at the virus and teaching the church to embrace all who seek its support. **INSIDE:** A bicycle ride built for AIDS awareness; the South is the new epicenter of the American AIDS epidemic, so why does federal funding still favor the North and West (**9**)? **PLUS:** Charting the age-old debate over when to start HIV treatment.

December

COVER: Sharon Stone's ability to get the rich and powerful involved in the search for the cure for HIV may help save our lives (**10**). **INSIDE:** POZ readers share how they survive AIDS in America; our annual guide to gift giving that benefits the HIV community. **PLUS:** Jon Benorden is fishing for answers—and awareness—in Alaska.

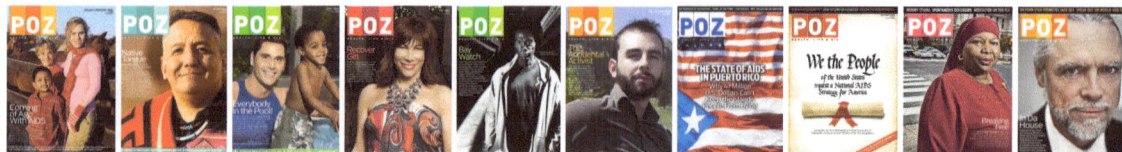

2008

January/February

COVER: Kentucky siblings Yonas, Mitchell and Alee were all born with HIV—and encouraged their mother, Suzan Stirling, to share their family's story. **INSIDE:** Four youth living with HIV share their strategies for a bold new generation of activism; how to talk to kids about sex when you're HIV positive. **PLUS:** Annie Lennox releases the AIDS anthem "Sing" to promote awareness (**1**).

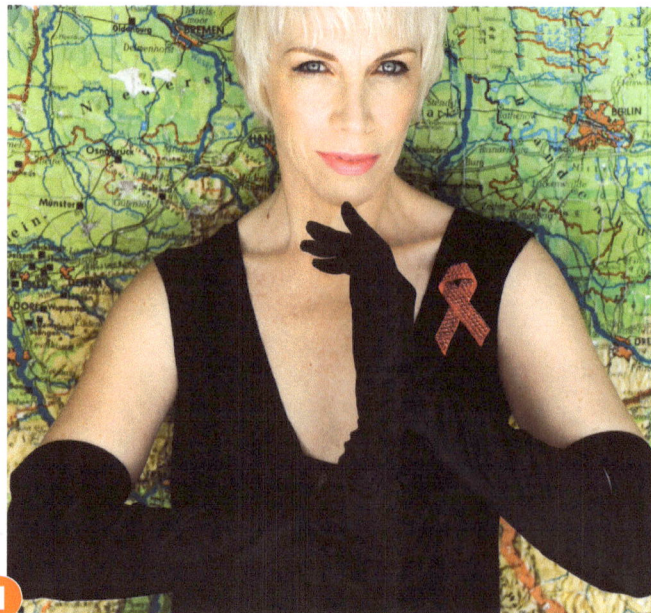

March

COVER: After being rejected by his Apache family, Kory Montoya became an advocate for the Native American HIV community (**2**). **INSIDE:** Why long-haul truckers are at risk for HIV; a snapshot of Art in a Box, a program that assists in recovery and empowerment through art. **PLUS:** Safety tips for preventing MRSA, a staph infection resistant to some antibiotics.

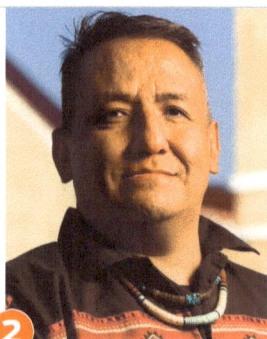

April

COVER: Toddler Caleb Glover became a poster child against discrimination after he was kicked out of a public swimming pool; champion swimmer and fashion designer Jack Mackenroth brings HIV awareness to *Project Runway* (**3**). **INSIDE:** Author Randy Boyd reflects on living with HIV for half his life. **PLUS:** Kiss rocker Gene Simmons represents the Elizabeth Glaser Pediatric AIDS Foundation on *Celebrity Apprentice*.

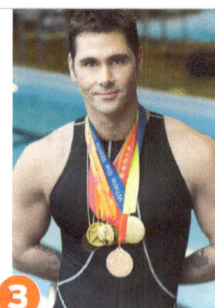

May

COVER: The rise, fall and rebound of former pop star Sherri Lewis. **INSIDE:** India's sex workers have curbed the rise of HIV through outreach, peer education and solidarity (**4**); a tribute to Oscar-nominated actor Denholm Elliott, best known for playing Dr. Marcus Brody in *Raiders of the Lost Ark*. **PLUS:** How to complement meds with alternative therapies.

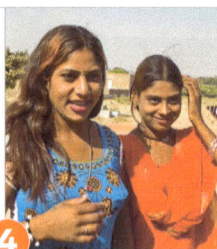

June

COVER: Kehn Coleman lives in Oakland, where HIV-positive residents fight for AIDS money and access to care, unlike some across the bay in San Francisco (**5**). **INSIDE:** After losing his family to AIDS-related illnesses, former Sergeant Ozzy Ramos creates a space for families to heal; New York City's Harlem United commemorates 20 years of serving the HIV community. **PLUS:** Porn goddess Chi Chi LaRue urges a boycott of barebacking videos.

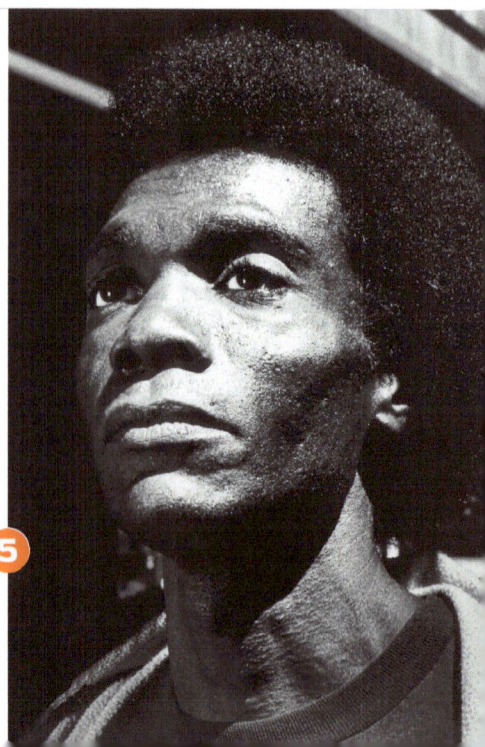

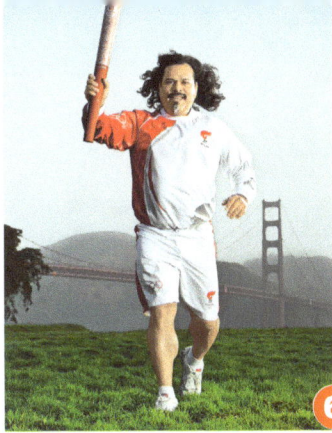

July/August

COVER: Peace Corps volunteer Jeremiah Johnson fights back after getting kicked out for testing positive during his service. **INSIDE:** Why migrants making the journey to the United States are at risk for HIV; an Olympic torchbearer living with HIV reflects on carrying the flame (**6**). **PLUS:** Debunking myths about the President's Emergency Plan for AIDS Relief (PEPFAR).

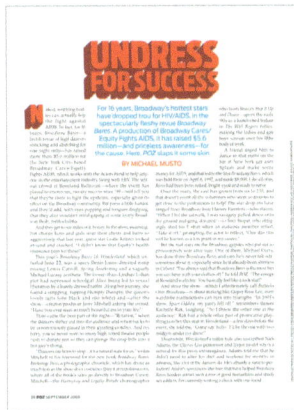
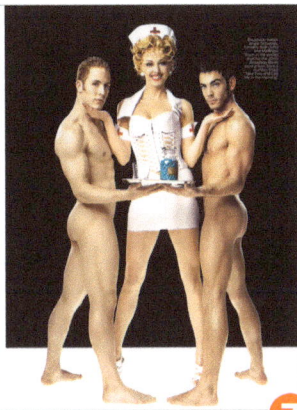

September

COVER: The sad state of AIDS resources in Puerto Rico. **INSIDE:** Michael Musto on *Broadway Bares*, the annual fleshy revue that raises money for Broadway Cares/Equity Fights AIDS (**7**); Iris House, an organization created to revolutionize AIDS services with programs that address the whole health of women living with HIV, turns 15. **PLUS:** Tips for dealing with nausea.

November

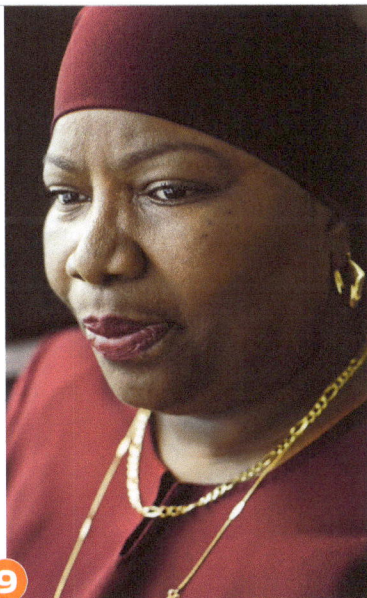

COVER: Ex-prisoner Waheedah Shabazz-El is now an AIDS educator for those behind bars (**9**). **INSIDE:** Shawn Decker explains his passion for beauty pageants; how to disclose in the heat of the moment. **PLUS:** *General Hospital*'s HIV-positive character, Dr. Robin Scorpio, is having a baby.

October

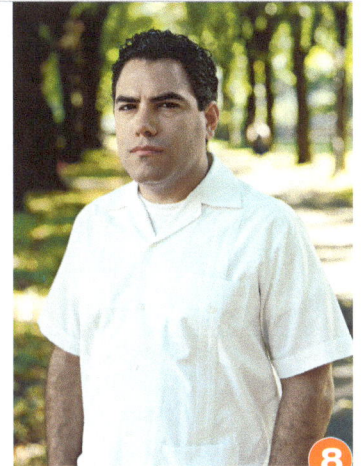

COVER: The HIV community in the United States wants a National AIDS Strategy. **INSIDE:** Kevin Fenton, director of National HIV/AIDS, Viral Hepatitis, STD and TB Prevention at the Centers for Disease Control and Prevention, discusses the latest figures for HIV/AIDS.

PLUS: POZ's new deputy editor, Oriol R. Gutierrez Jr., shares how he came out twice to his family—first as gay and again as HIV positive (**8**).

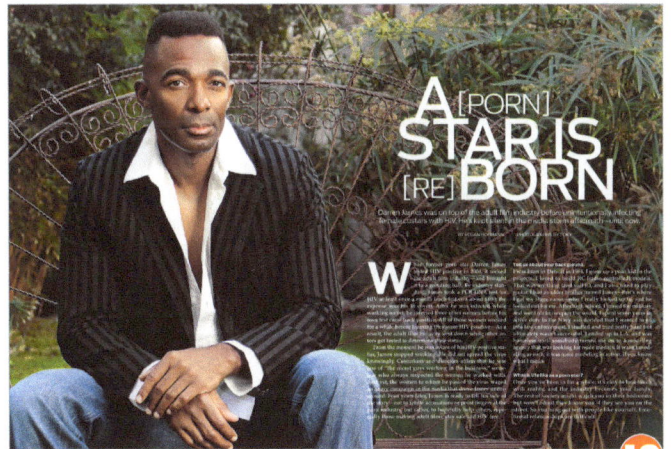

December

COVER: Housing Works CEO Charles King is a champion for housing for the homeless as a form of HIV prevention. **INSIDE:** Porn star Darren James opens up after unintentionally transmitting HIV to female costars in 2004 (**10**); holiday gifts that give back. **PLUS:** The POZ and AIDSmeds drug chart compares available medication options.

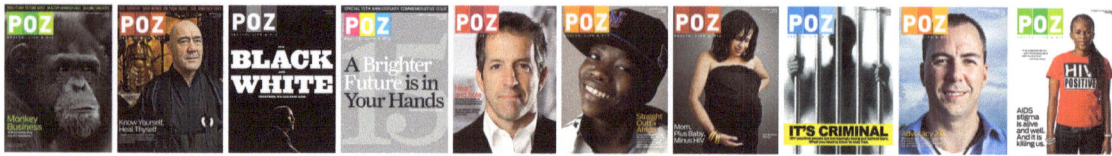

2009

January/February

COVER: Jethro, a chimpanzee that spent years in a lab and was used for HIV research, was released to a chimp sanctuary in Canada. **INSIDE:** POZ asks Kevin Frost, CEO of amfAR, The Foundation for AIDS Research whether it pays to cure AIDS (**1**). **PLUS:** A biopic about MTV's Pedro Zamora.

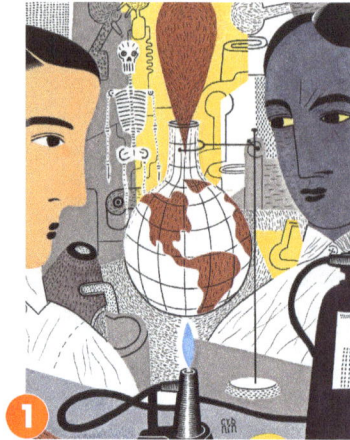

March

COVER: Robert "Chodo" Campbell, a Buddhist monk living with HIV, shows us how to live well in the moment—and for a lifetime of tomorrows (**2**). **INSIDE:** When foreign tourists connect with local sex workers, both are often at risk. **PLUS:** People living with HIV in the United States are taking flight for better, cheaper facial fillers (**3**).

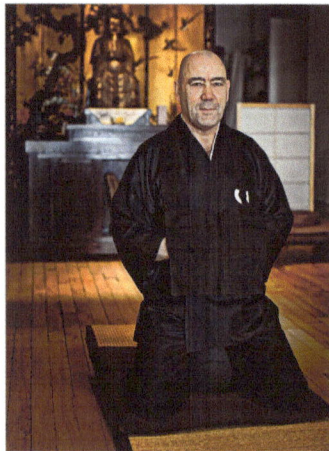

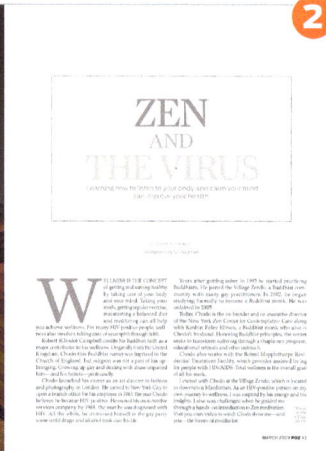

April

COVER: Will President Barack Obama herald in a new era of health care (**4**)? **INSIDE:** Info on how to lobby Congress for AIDS programs; a chart of who's who when it comes to federal oversight of HIV funding. **PLUS:** An ode to the late activist Martin Delaney, founder of Project Inform.

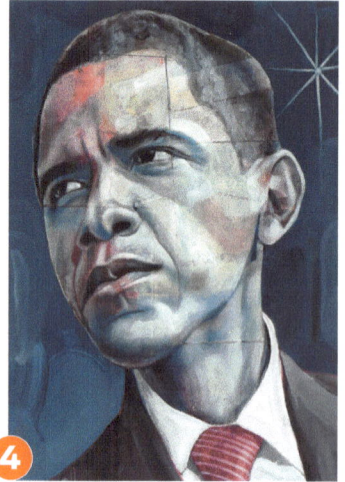

May

COVER: The 15th anniversary of POZ. **INSIDE:** A look at some of the defining moments in the magazine's history; several people share how their disclosure of HIV in the pages of POZ changed their lives; an abbreviated encyclopedia of AIDS; portraits of a community fighting stigma. **PLUS:** Founder Sean Strub reflects on the magazine's origin—and his next move (**5**).

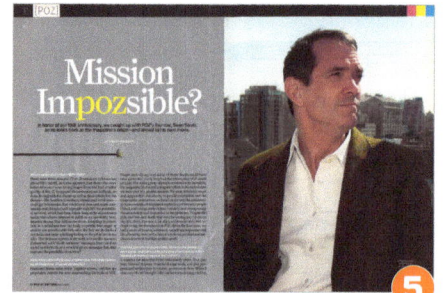

June

COVER: Fashion designer Kenneth Cole uses his advertising campaigns to sell shoes, belts, handbags and clothes—while raising awareness of social issues, including AIDS. **INSIDE:** Rachel Maddow, host of her eponymous MSNBC show, has been an avid AIDS activist for years—and now addresses HIV on prime-time TV (**6**). **PLUS:** Lesbians living with HIV.

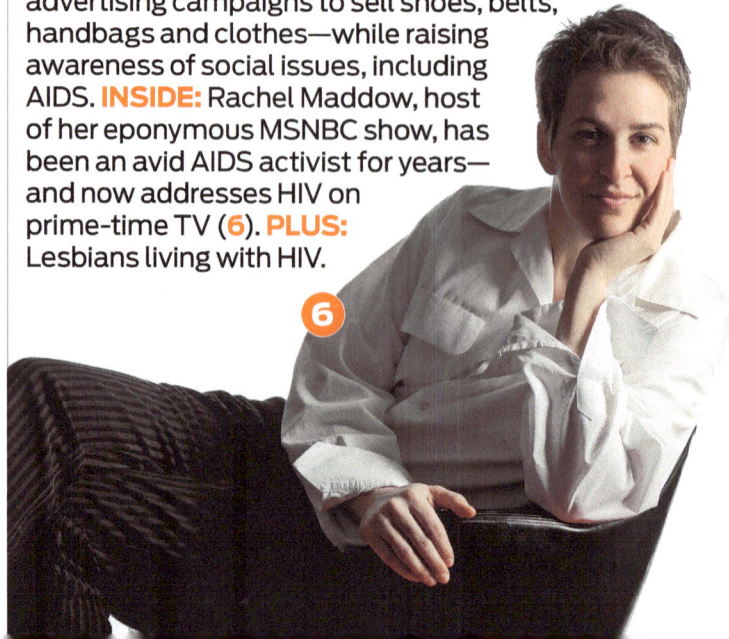

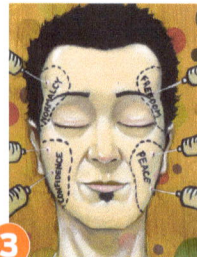

July/August

COVER: Noah Mushimiyimana, a Rwandan rapper, lost his innocence to AIDS yet regained his swagger thanks to Keep a Child Alive and *American Idol* (**7**).
INSIDE: A peek into photographer Kristen Ashburn's new book about AIDS in Africa, *I Am Because We Are*.
PLUS: Looking at the promise—and the price—of treatment as prevention.

September

COVER: Luz de Jesus Roman is a Latina mom living with HIV who invites POZ along on her journey of having an HIV-negative baby girl (**8**).
INSIDE: Keeping AIDS at bay in Cuba; the media should pay attention to Latinos living with HIV; *Our Bodies, Ourselves* devotes an entire chapter to HIV/AIDS.
PLUS: A collection of first-person narratives of African-American gay men in the South is "serving tea."

October

COVER: People living with HIV are increasingly being put behind bars. What you need to know to stay free. **INSIDE:** An excerpt from *I Have Something to Tell You*, a memoir by POZ editor-in-chief Regan Hofmann (**9**); challenging the media to raise HIV awareness. **PLUS:** Why condoms shouldn't be locked up (**10**).

November

COVER: Michael Emanuel Rajner, an HIV activist living with the virus, represents a new breed of AIDS advocate. **INSIDE:** Welcome to AIDS Advocacy 2.0, a new era of activism (**11**); rapid at-home HIV testing is inching closer to reality. **PLUS:** How you can be an AIDS advocate.

December

COVER: Nokhwezi Hoboyi, an HIV-positive activist from the Treatment Action Campaign in South Africa, bears witness to AIDS stigma. **INSIDE:** Seth Berkley of the International AIDS Vaccine Initiative talks about vaccine research; comic book creator Darren Davis is doing super, despite HIV. **PLUS:** Portraits from *Infected & Affected* by Joan Lobis Brown (**12**).

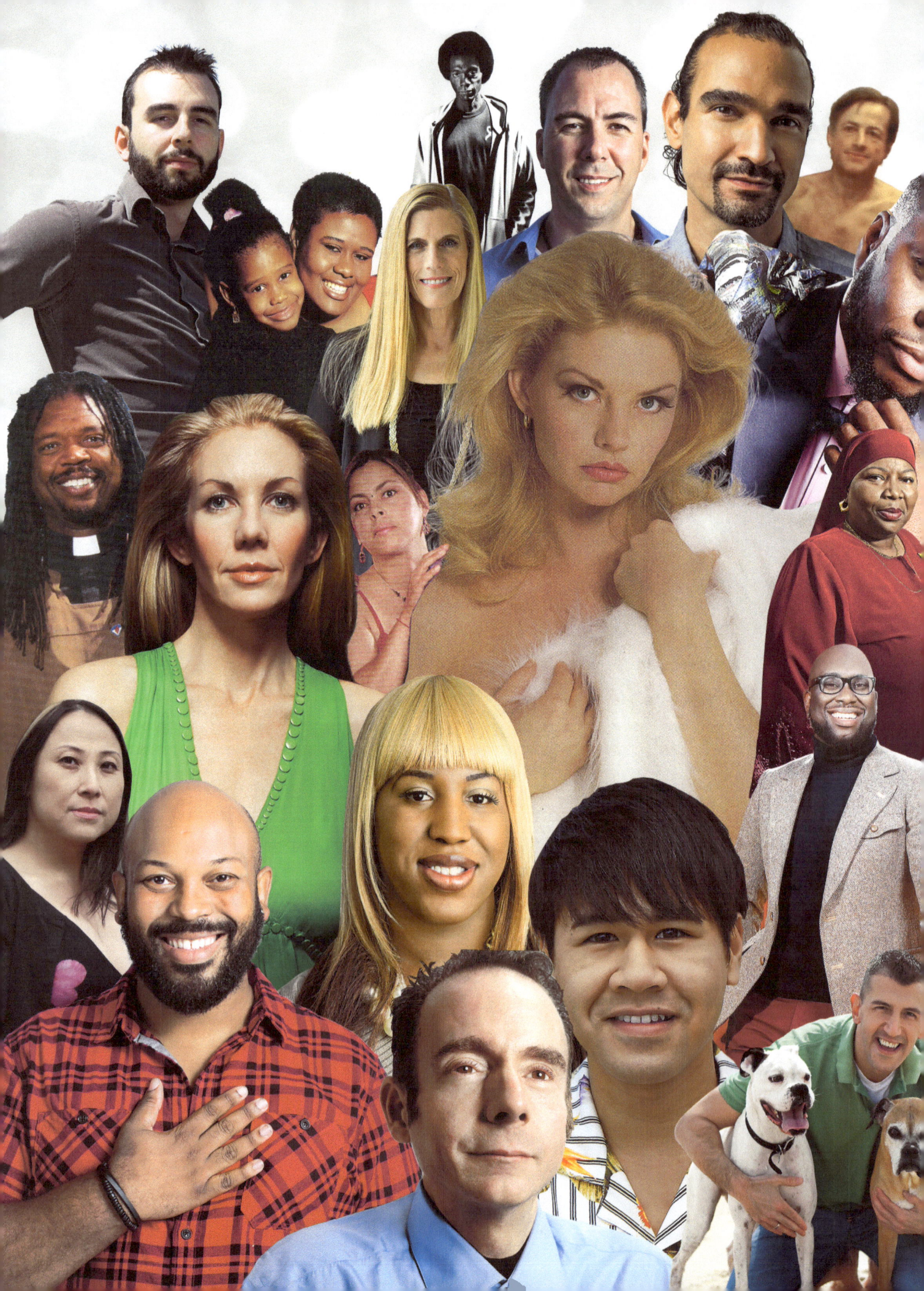

25 Years of Advocates

TWENTY-FIVE ADVOCATES SHARE WHAT POZ MEANS TO THEM.

BY CASEY HALTER AND TIM MURPHY

When *POZ debuted in* 1994, effective HIV treatment didn't exist. That wouldn't come to pass until two years later. The successful launch 25 years ago of a magazine for people living with HIV/AIDS was, to say the least, not assured. And yet, despite all the naysayers and challenges, POZ has endured.

Recounting the magazine's mission in his 2014 memoir, *Body Counts*, POZ founder Sean Strub writes, "We tried to tell the story of the

Images of the 25 advocates as they appeared in POZ

epidemic in all its complexities, through the experience of those with HIV. And we would do so in an attractive, engaging, and hopeful format. On glossy paper."

From the very beginning, POZ has strived to live up to that mission every day, in print and online—from fighting for effective treatment to advocating for the expansion of access to that treatment, from diminishing the fear of people living with HIV to promoting the fact that being undetectable means not being able to transmit the virus sexually.

Over the years, readers have shared

with us how much they value POZ in their lives. We are humbled by the praise and take seriously the responsibility of serving the HIV community. For a few readers, however, being spotlighted on the cover of the magazine has had an even deeper effect.

For some, being on the cover supercharged their advocacy. For others, the cover confirmed that their advocacy had made a difference. For all of them, appearing in POZ marked a milestone in their lives.

Here, we honor 25 of these advocates. We thank them—and all of you—for continuing to support POZ.

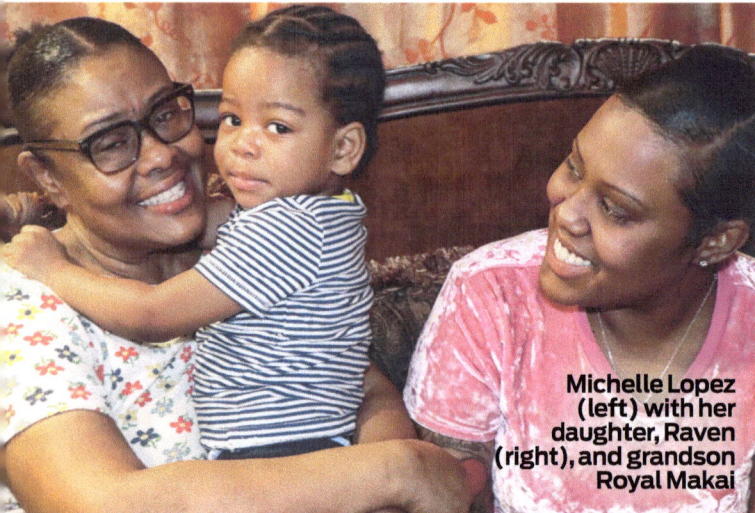

Michelle Lopez (left) with her daughter, Raven (right), and grandson Royal Makai

Michelle and Raven Lopez

"I remember going to a park in the Bronx and the photographer telling my mother to put me in the swing and put her face next to mine."

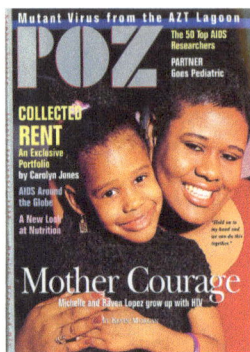

That's how Raven, 28, remembers her 1996 POZ cover shoot. She was 5 years old, and her well-known HIV activist mom, Michelle, posed with her to show the world that both an HIV-positive mom and child could lead happy and healthy lives with the virus—even in what was then only year 1 of the era of highly effective antiretroviral treatment for the virus.

"That cover led me to come out publicly with my HIV status later in life," says Raven, who still lives with her mom in Brooklyn. "I even met and became friends with [fellow HIV-positive POZ cover kid] Hydeia Broadbent. We have the same birthday."

Raven is studying to become a phlebotomist and is the proud mother of an HIV-negative 2-year-old son, Royal Makai. Of course, that also means Michelle, 52, is a proud grandma—and, as ever, a fiercely outspoken HIV activist, currently consulting for GMHC/ACRIA on issues of HIV in women over 50. "My program's going to be called Pussy Talk 50, all about our sexual health," she declares.

Lest you think such talk embarrasses Raven, she has this to say about her mom: "She's taught me how to become a strong, independent woman. That's why I'm comfortable talking about my status with anyone—even on a date." And, she says, when uninformed men tell her she looks too sexy to have HIV, she just shows them her POZ cover!

Rebekka Armstrong

Playboy magazine's Miss September 1986, Armstrong had gone public with her 1989 HIV diagnosis four years before she appeared on POZ's cover, but the bisexual bombshell, now 52, still remembers that "life-changing" moment.

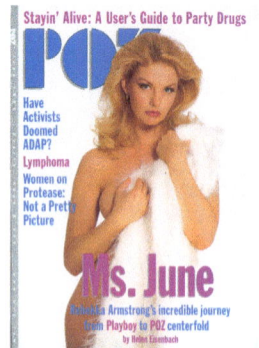

"For Playboy, I was showing you my body and some of my brains, but with POZ, I was actually showing the world who I was with a really intense purpose, which was empowering," she says. "People would come up to me and say, 'Oh my God, I had no idea you had AIDS' or 'This is what AIDS could look like.' It gave me a whole new platform to educate people."

She was also getting seriously sick at the time, but today, she says, she's in great health. "I've been sober 13 years now," says the former speed user.

Plus, Armstrong is in business with Buck Angel, the former porn actor she calls her "chosen dad," selling her own line of healing balms and tinctures containing cannabidiol (CBD) oil produced by and with Angel's business PrideWellness.net. A portion of all sales are donated to AIDS service organizations.

A former professional bodybuilder, Armstrong is now a personal trainer and sports therapy aide who, despite having had shoulder surgery, still lifts weights—though they're lighter these days. She spends much of the rest of her time walking her four rescue dogs in the hills of Los Angeles with concert rigger Anthony DiSpirito, her partner of 11 years. "He's the love of my life," she says.

Oh, and she's still looking sexy on those massive AIDS Healthcare Foundation billboards in LA. "Thriving," they read. And is she ever.

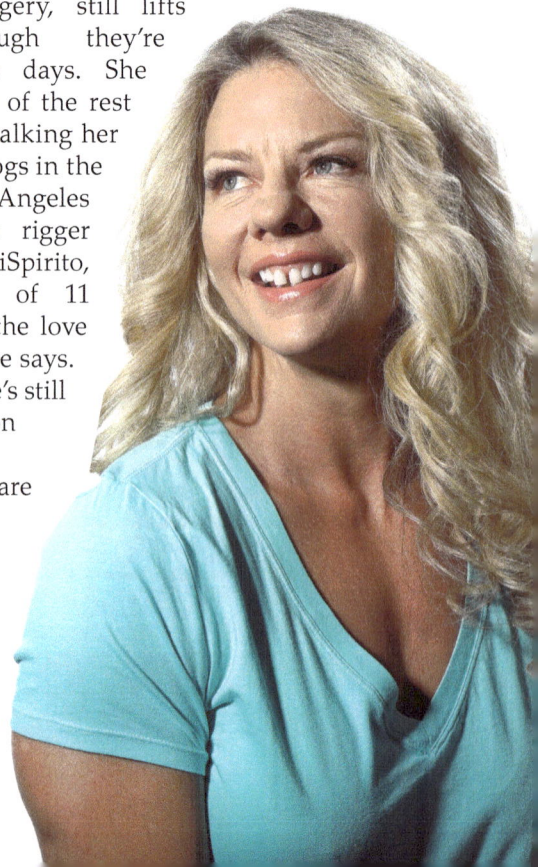

(LOPEZ, CHEEKS, RODRIGUEZ) COURTESY OF INDIVIDUALS, (ARMSTRONG) COURTESY OF AIDS HEALTHCARE FOUNDATION

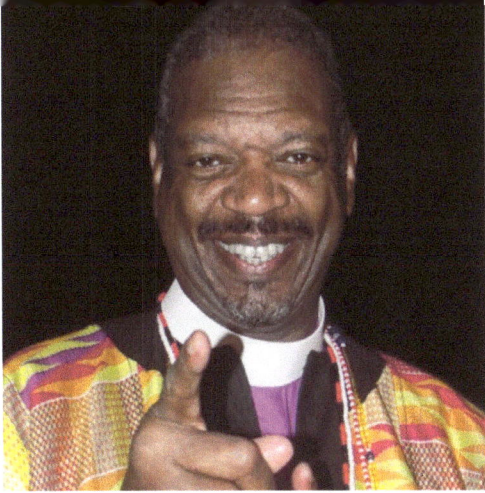

PREVIOUS PAGES: (ARMSTRONG) CAROLYN JONES, (BROWN) TOBY BURDITT, (CHEEKS) D.A. PETERSON, (CHUNG) JEFF SINGER, (COLEMAN) IAN MARTIN, (FLEURY/MALAVE) SCOTT PASFIELD, (HOFMANN) JACK LOUTH, (HORN) KEVIN MCDERMOTT, (HOWARD) JONATHAN TIMMES, (JOHNSON) DAN CHAVKIN, (KING AND TERRY) JONATHAN TIMMES, (J. LEWIS, O. LEWIS, MUÑOZ, SANCHEZ AND SHABAZZ-EL) BILL WADMAN, (M. LOPEZ, R. LOPEZ) JOHN BONDELLIO, (MORELLET) ANDREW EINHORN, (RAINER) BRIAN SMITH, (RODRIGUEZ) ROBIN HOLLAND, (TIN) ARI MICHELSON, (WOODS) LYNN LANE

Bishop Kwabena Rainier "Rainey" Cheeks

"I was surprised by how people responded to it," says Cheeks. That's how the Washington, DC–based founder of the pioneering Black gay AIDS agency Us Helping Us and the LGBT-affirming Inner Light Unity Fellowship Church remembers his POZ cover appearance 20 years ago.

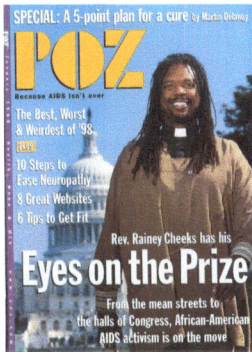

"I thought I was very public with my status, but many people who knew me thought it was quite bold of me." He says it also helped with fundraising and landing more speaking engagements. "Having that kind of national exposure was a powerful thing."

In 1999, Cheeks, now 66, had already been living with HIV for several years. He remains the pastor of Inner Light, which celebrated its 25th anniversary last year, and is looking forward to hosting more workshops and seminars to empower gay Black men, who still have the highest HIV rates in the United States. "I do a workshop called 'The Arc of Loving Yourself.' How can we gay men respect, and not objectify, each other?"

In recent years, he has worked extensively to try to get mainline churches to become LGBT-affirming. "I started my meetings with all of them by asking, 'Tell me who's not welcome to the table of God?'" The result? A bunch of ministers held a service during which they stood in the pulpit and apologized to their LGBT churchgoers for not having explicitly embraced them in the past.

When Cheeks, the author of *Reclaiming Your Divine Birthright*, isn't working, he hikes in Rock Creek Park, participates in an African drumming circle and enjoys time with his beloved collection of elephant figurines. "Elephants are family," he explains. "They take care of one another."

Susan Rodriguez

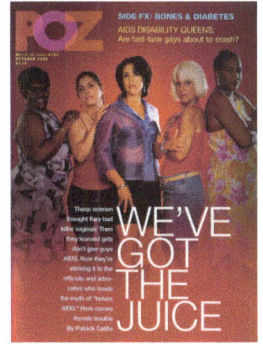

Rodriguez, 59, originally appeared on the cover of POZ in 1997 for a story about folks with HIV quitting their jobs and going on benefits to take care of themselves.

That first cover "played a major role in shaping my life and activism," she says—so much so that she went on to found SMART (Sisterhood Mobilized for AIDS/HIV Research & Treatment) University in New York City to provide support, education and advocacy for women living with HIV.

In the fall of 2001, she appeared on the cover again, flanked by four of her fellow SMART ladies, for a story about new data confirming that sexual transmission of HIV from women to men is rare in the United States. But her most vivid memory of that issue of POZ is that it came out on 9/11, after which SMART had to temporarily vacate its downtown Manhattan offices as a result of the wreckage and pollution from the terrorist attack. "A sense of hopelessness set in [during] the days and weeks afterward," she recalls. "Continuing SMART became my focal point to get out of despair."

And Rodriguez has done so to this day. She recently started SMART HEART, which fuses activism and creativity for women with HIV via sign-making parties for protests and a meditation/healing component. "Our participants are primarily low-income women of color, and we felt that it was important to build a foundation of civic engagement leading to the midterm elections and now beyond," she says. A breast cancer, stroke and depression survivor, she adds, "It's important that I keep my life balanced and take care of myself mentally and physically."

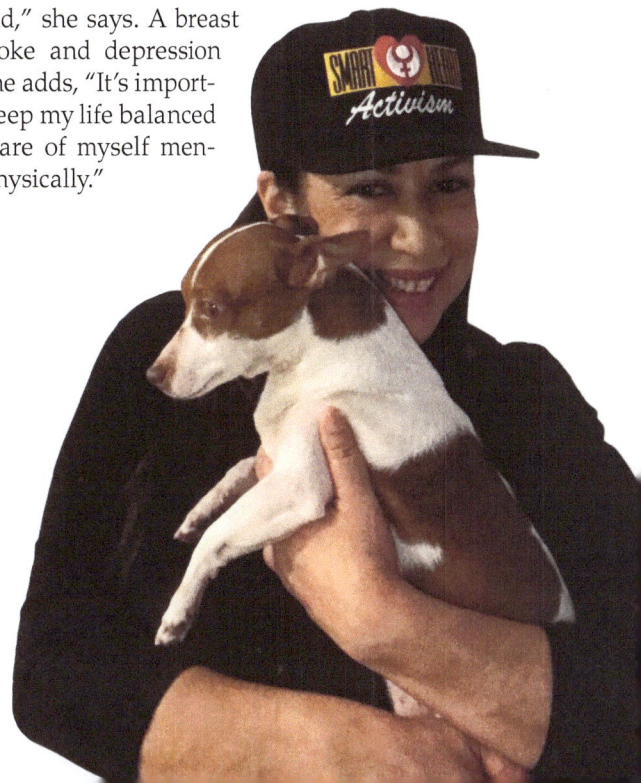

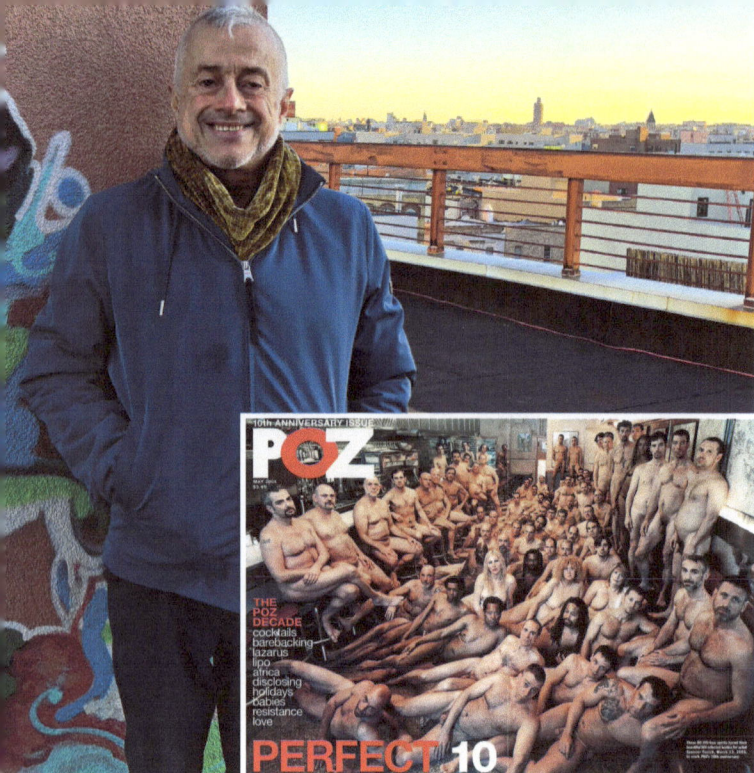

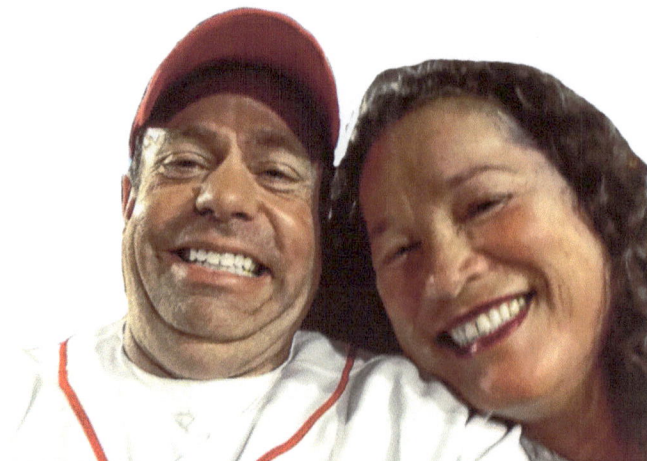

FEBRUARY/MARCH 2006

Bryan Fleury and Millie Malave

Fleury appeared on the cover of POZ with the love of his life and fellow advocate Malave. Both say their romance is stronger today than ever. "Being in the magazine was the first time either of us went public [about living with HIV] and was the greatest decision we ever made," says Fleury, an HIV prevention educator who lives in Massachusetts.

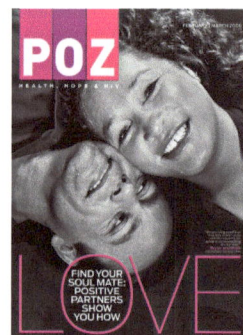

The article told the stories of five couples—both positive and negative—who found love in the face of HIV. "It gave so many people hope that true love exists, plus we were one of the very first heterosexual couples put on the cover," Fleury says proudly.

To this day, he says his love story is a staple of his sex-ed curriculum in schools. His advice for keeping the flame alive all these years? "Keep yourself undetectable, adhere to your meds, enjoy a happy sex life," he jokes.

"Even though I live in New York," says Malave, "Bryan and I take turns traveling back and forth to Massachusetts to be with each other." As was the case for Fleury, Malave's decision to appear on the cover was an easy one. "I wanted other HIV-positive people to know that they also can find love after HIV."

Malave, a former nurse, has traveled the world with Fleury, setting sail on five cruises tailored to people living with HIV. Unlike her boyfriend, Malave isn't as vocal about living with HIV in her everyday life but still considers herself an advocate. "My role has been mostly trying to stay healthy for my three daughters," says Malave.

The couple recently took a big new step in their relationship when they adopted two rescue dogs. "They give me such unconditional love," says Millie, "but, most importantly, I just enjoy being alive and being with my family."

MAY 2004

Florent Morellet

POZ's 10th anniversary cover garnered global attention after famed artist Spencer Tunick created an installation of 80 naked men and women living with HIV—some of them now deceased—one frigid early morning in New York's Meatpacking District.

The setting? Florent, the longtime beloved bohemian diner and onetime POZ magazine unofficial canteen, which closed in 2008. Its namesake proprietor is the iconic HIV-positive French activist, artist and provocateur Florent Morellet, who was known to track his T cells on the diner's letterboards alongside the menu. He also attended the photo shoot.

Morellet, 65, now lives in Bushwick, an arty Brooklyn neighborhood with a vibe that echoes that of his diner's 1980s and '90s heyday. "It was fantastic," he remembers of the cover image. "I think it was one of the restaurant's greatest moments. People called me about it from all over the world. It was political and sensational—but with humor. It was a wonderful reminder that so many of us had survived together, as a family, up to that point."

Morellet lives a much quieter life these days. "It's difficult to be retired and not be at the center of the world anymore." Not completely separated from his past, he's still good friends with his ex, the novelist Peter Cameron.

In 2018, Morellet moved longtime Florent employee Harry Eriksen into his apartment and coordinated Eriksen's hospice care. Eriksen died of cancer in November. "He was my right hand at the restaurant and my soul mate," says Morellet. "People tell me they're sorry, but, actually, he died in my arms, and it was one of the most beautiful things in my life."

Regan Hofmann

Hofmann had been writing an anonymous column for POZ ("In the Closet") about living secretly with HIV for a few years before she became editor-in-chief of the magazine. She came out with a splash, not just on our cover but also in the pages of Vogue, New York magazine and The New York Times. (All that was followed by her 2009 memoir, *I Have Something to Tell You*.)

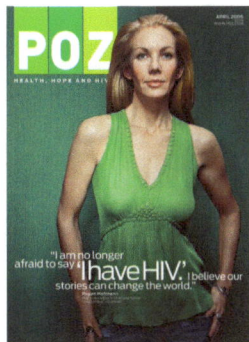

As POZ's first HIV-positive editor-in-chief, the stylish, horse-riding Hofmann brought new attention to the magazine during her six-year tenure, often appearing in gowns on red carpets for HIV galas for groups such as amfAR, The Foundation for AIDS Research. Her passion for finding the cure led her to joining amfAR's board.

"Being on the cover of POZ, while initially terrifying, was the most liberating, empowering thing I have done," she says. "I lived in emotional isolation for nearly 10 years, keeping my HIV status a secret from most people. Telling my truth publicly felt like being born again—into a huge family of people just like me."

Currently, Hofmann is the policy officer of the Joint United Nations Programme on HIV/AIDS (UNAIDS) Liaison Office in Washington, DC, where she works with the U.S. government "to encourage continued strong bipartisan American leadership on AIDS." She also supports UNAIDS executive leadership and country teams in their work around the world.

The former New Jersey girl now lives on a small farm outside DC with her beloved horse and her Muscovy ducks. "Which," she points out, "I raise for eggs, not meat!"

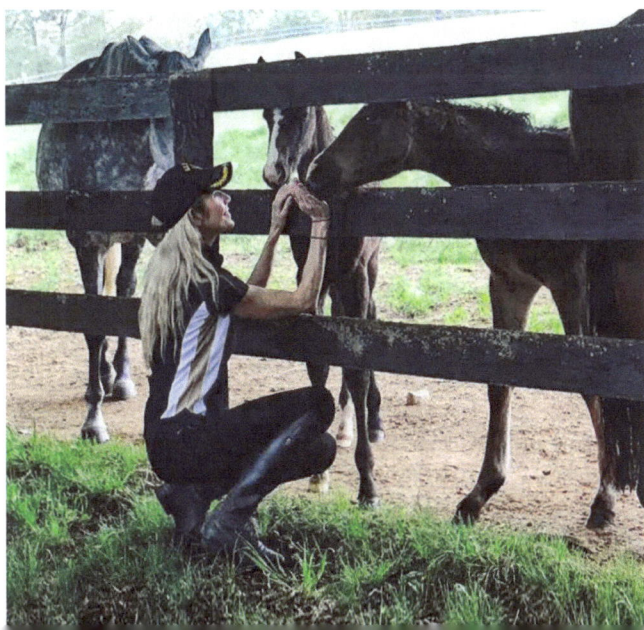

Kehn Coleman

"Things are a lot different since I did that interview," says Coleman, when asked about the time he appeared on the cover of POZ. The article addressed the incredible difference in HIV care between San Francisco and Oakland, two California cities separated by just eight miles—and decades of racial and socioeconomic disparities.

"At that time, I was not working yet. I had just finished my associate's degree and was looking for something positive to give back," he says. A survivor of not just HIV but also of homelessness, Coleman was one of many people struggling to find care who were profiled for the article.

Today, Coleman has a job assisting special-needs children in San Francisco, a post he has held proudly since 2009. "It's my way of giving back," says the quiet advocate, uncle and educator, who has been living with HIV since 1993. "I feel as though I've been given so many options as a long-term survivor. I figure sometimes that I've been given a chance to survive to help others."

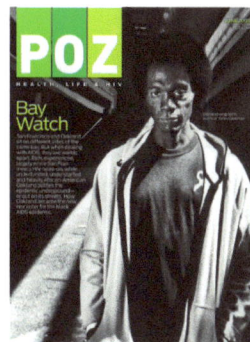

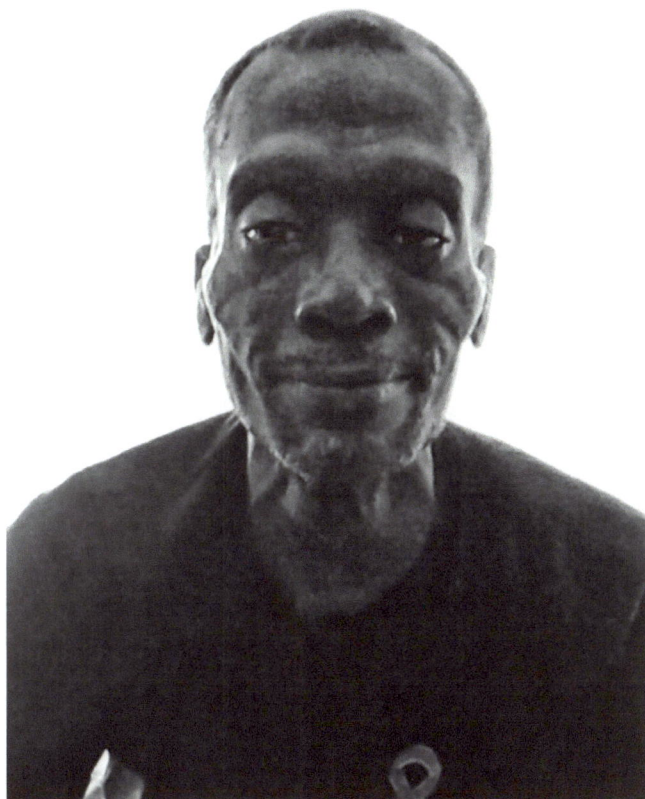

Jeremiah Johnson

Shortly after Johnson, 36, appeared on the cover of POZ to protest being sent home from Ukraine by the Peace Corps because he tested HIV positive, another foreign aid organization saw the magazine and reached out to him, offering him a similar position in Lima, Peru. But in addition to that concrete outcome, "being on the cover was transformative for me," he says. "It elevated my activism and contributed to my resilience, because I was in a state of shock at my dismissal."

It was this resilience that led him, with the American Civil Liberties Union (ACLU) and POZ, to successfully pressure the Peace Corps to end its policy of sending members home for testing positive for the by-then easily treatable virus. (Unfortunately, that policy has recently reemerged; see Romany Tin on page 84.)

At the time of the cover shoot, Johnson was depressed and waiting tables back in his native Denver. But since then, he has thrived as a person and an activist. Since 2011, he has lived in New York, where he was recently promoted to HIV project director at the venerable think tank Treatment Action Group. He also played a large role after the 2016 election in founding the ACT UP–like direct-action collective Rise and Resist, whose members have been arrested several times while protesting President Trump and the policies of the right-wing 115th Congress.

Johnson is in a long-term relationship with dancer and massage therapist Tym Byers, who joins him for work conferences. And he says much of his current activism can be traced back to that POZ cover. "With my face suddenly out there," he says, "it helped me get around any inhibitions I had about being public and able to talk about discrimination and stigma openly."

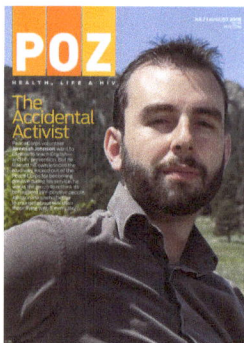

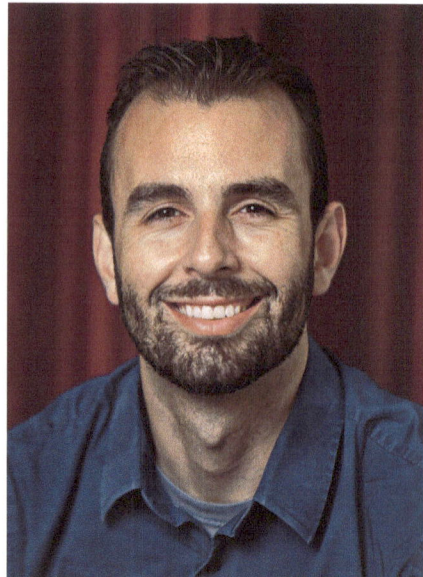

Waheedah Shabazz-El

"To this day, people still remember me from the cover of POZ magazine," says Waheedah Shabazz-El, HIV survivor, mother of three, grandmother of four and outspoken advocate in America's Muslim, LGBT and Black communities. "I've had the opportunity to speak a lot since then, and I'll still wear the same garment," she says. "When I do that, I'm like: 'You're getting it all today, you know!'"

Back then, Shabazz-El was just starting to share her HIV diagnosis, which she received while in jail in 2003. She has since catapulted into a renowned advocacy career working with the likes of ACT UP Philadelphia, Positive Women's Network–USA, Women of Color United Against Violence and HIV, CHAMP and the Philadelphia Network of Care for Prisoner Reentry in her hometown of Philly, among many others.

Today, her fight is about more than just a serostatus. "All my advocacy was around HIV," Shabazz-El recalls. "Now, my advocacy is around human rights. Over the years, I've had the opportunity to see things that have increased my awareness and broadened my perspective. There are intersecting oppressions."

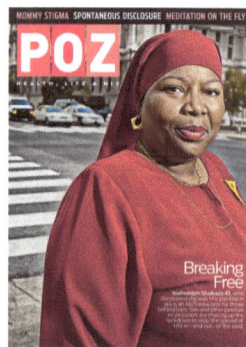

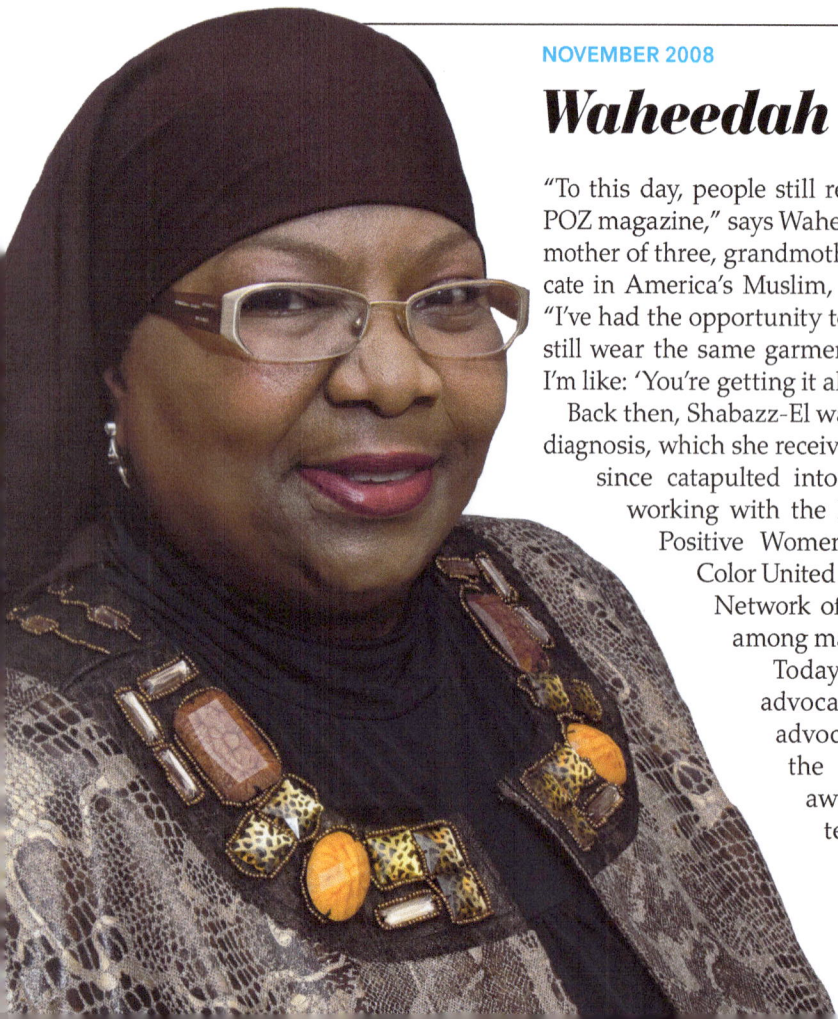

NOVEMBER 2009

Michael Emanuel Rajner

As the legislative director of the Florida Gay, Lesbian, Bisexual and Transgender Democratic Caucus, Rajner was constantly emailing POZ to feed editors tips for potential stories and to ask whether anyone on staff wanted to press presidential candidates on AIDS. That was in 2009.

"But around and leading up to 2016, I stepped away more and more from engaging with HIV/AIDS issues," Rajner explains. "I'm now going on 25 years living with HIV, and I think that a shift has been happening. Minority communities are finally having greater opportunities to have their voices heard, and people like me have had to step back so others can step up and have that opportunity."

But that doesn't mean the former policy powerhouse has gone completely silent. Last year, Rajner connected with students from Parkland, Florida, to share old-school HIV activism advice after they stepped into advocacy following one of the deadliest school shootings in U.S. history.

"Activism doesn't mean you have to be attending a conference or be the person on the front line," says Rajner. "Sometimes it's more important to be available to people as a resource or to help guide new people who are stepping forward. And that's what I'm trying to do."

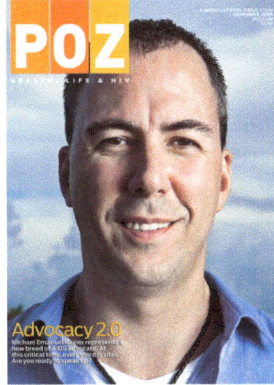

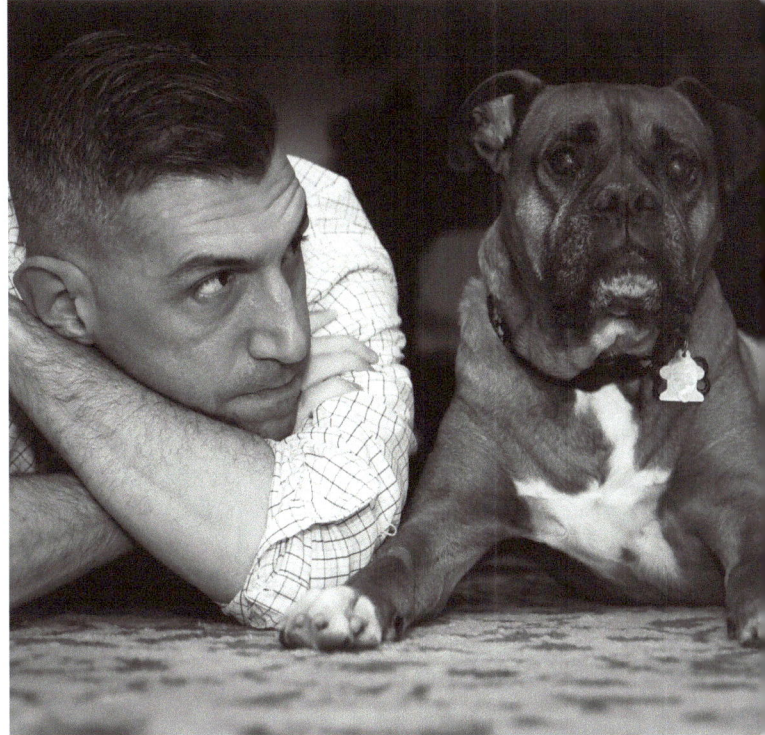

(RAJNER, HORN) COURTESY OF INDIVIDUALS

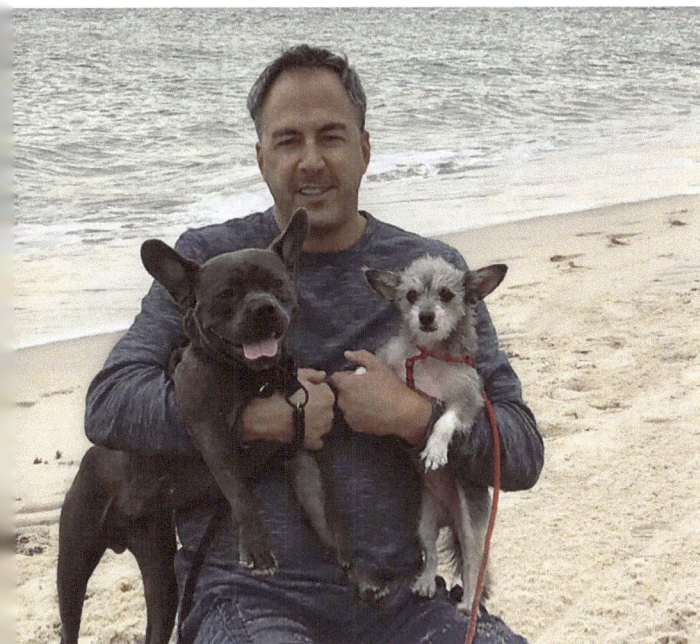

JUNE 2010

Tim Horn

Horn's history with POZ goes way back. "I authored its first feature on the development and launch of protease inhibitors," he recalls. He then went on to edit Physicians' Research Network Notebook, a quarterly magazine for HIV care providers, and POZ sister site AIDSmeds.com before helping to lead the Treatment Action Group for several years as a writer and activist.

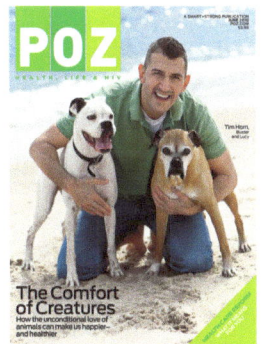

Needless to say, a lot has changed both for him and in HIV research since those early days. "It's weird to think of HIV as a 'career,' but it has been at the center of my work for my entire adult life thus far," says Horn, who currently works on HIV prevention and treatment access for the National Alliance of State and Territorial AIDS Directors (NASTAD).

Horn's cover story was about the countless ways our four-legged companions keep us happy and healthy. He remains an animal lover but has expanded his interests. "I'm an amateur photographer and am attempting to tackle the dark arts of bread baking," says Horn. "I'm still here continuing the challenge of living my best life."

Timothy Ray Brown

By the time Brown, 53, was featured on the cover of POZ, he had already lived through about three years as the first person in the world known to have been cured of HIV.

Diagnosed with the virus in 1995, he was undergoing a stem-cell transplant for cancer in Germany in the 2000s when he agreed to let the doctor infuse him with cells harvested from a donor with a genetic mutation that blocked HIV. Brown has been HIV negative ever since.

Researchers are still a long way from transforming what Brown's extraordinary case taught us about HIV eradication into a workable large-scale cure.

Dubbed "the Berlin Patient" by global media because he was living in that city at the time, the Seattle native is back in the United States living happily and healthily—despite some neuropathy and joint stiffness—in Palm Springs, California, with his boyfriend, Tim Hoeffgen, and their cat, Penny.

He does yoga weekly, volunteers with the Desert AIDS Project to provide resources for locals struggling with meth addiction, including a potential needle-exchange site, and is involved in the area's HIV+Aging Research Project–Palm Springs (harp-ps.org).

He still regularly attends conferences about an HIV cure, including one in Seattle in early 2019, where researchers announced that a second man is in long-term HIV remission after a similar procedure.

"I think it's getting close to something that should be called a cure," Brown says. "I can't wait to meet him."

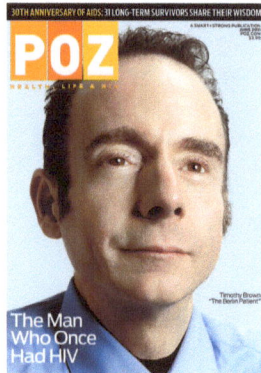

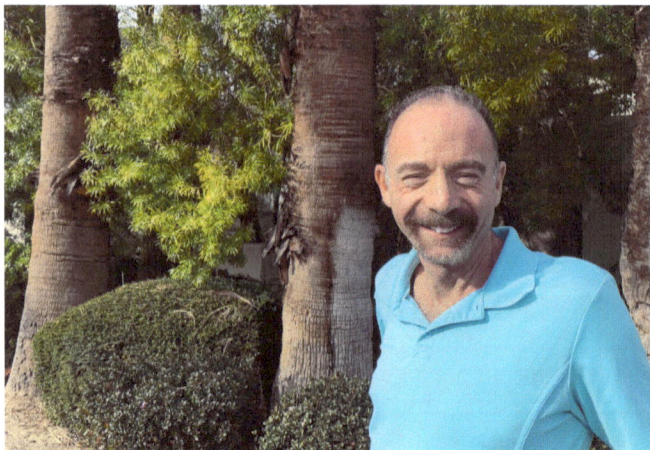

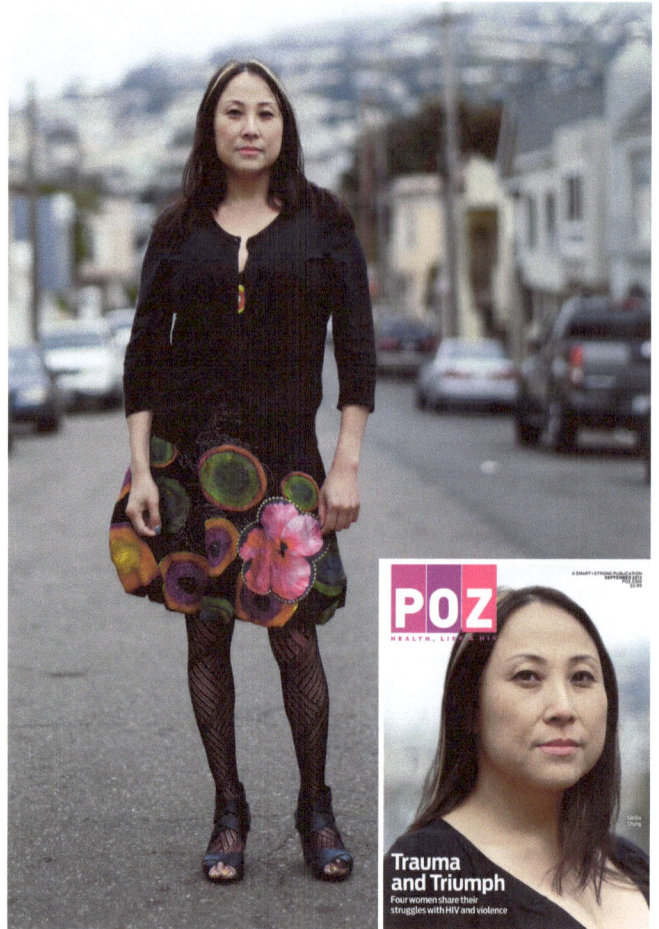

Cecilia Chung

"Things have changed since then, but they haven't changed that much," says Chung when asked about her 2012 POZ cover story. The article came out the same year the trans community noted a significant increase in violent attacks on trans women across the country, and advocates like Chung were looking to fight back.

"I had been visible for quite a while by that time," Chung recalls, adding that appearing on the cover seemed like a natural progression of her career as a positive trans activist. At the time, she was serving as a health commissioner in San Francisco, a post she still holds, and was a senior strategist at the Transgender Law Center, which remains the nation's largest trans-led advocacy organization.

In the past six years, "I've spent a lot of time nurturing the next generation of leaders," says Chung, who's ready to pass the torch after nearly 30 years of speaking out. "I really believe that in order for us to break down stigma, we have to be able to see others who look like us and who can share our stories."

JUNE 2013

Mark S. King

An LGBT advocate, King is the creator of the HIV blog My Fabulous Disease. But it wasn't until this cover story, which he penned, that he saw himself as a writer. "That article changed the way people viewed me, and it changed the opportunities that I got in terms of being able to speak out as a person living with HIV," he says.

Since then, the blogger/activist has written about crystal meth addiction as a gay man; U.S. HIV politics; iconic AIDS history; why there are still about 7,000 AIDS-related deaths each year in the United States; and more. His byline has appeared in such outlets as The Advocate, Newsweek, Queerty and TheBody.com.

"As a writer, activist and long-term survivor, I view every opportunity to share my voice on the pages of POZ as a privilege and something I consider to be an important piece of my legacy," he says. Find him online, on social media and in future issues of POZ magazine.

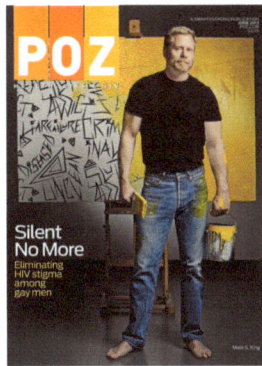

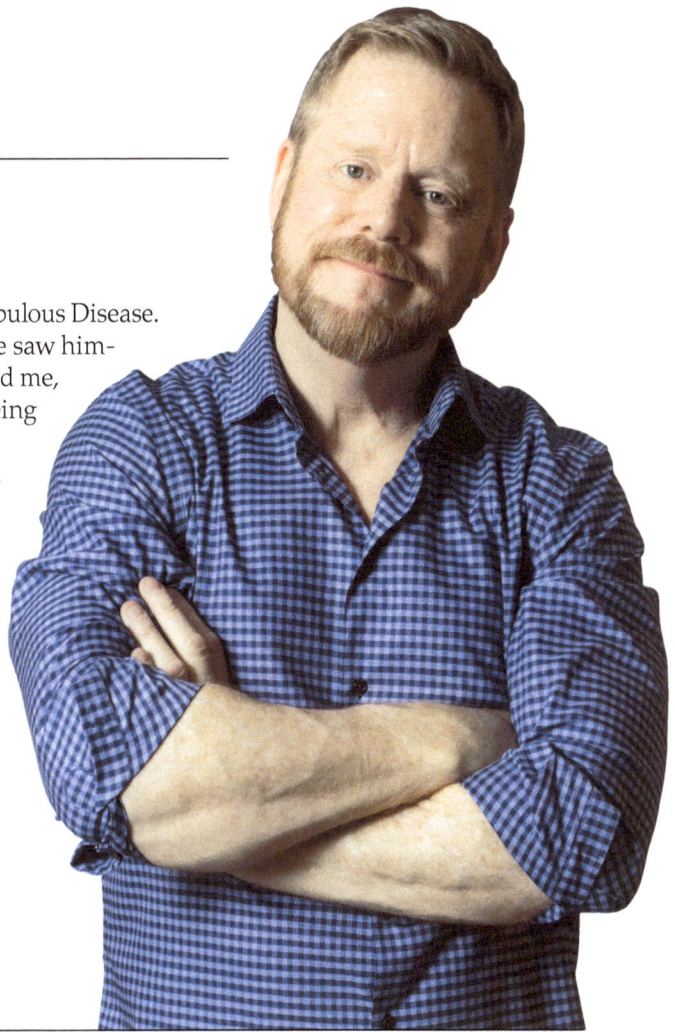

SEPTEMBER 2014

Julie Lewis (left) with her son Ryan

Julie Lewis

Diagnosed with HIV in 1990 after contracting the virus via a 1984 blood transfusion, Lewis—the mother of Macklemore's musical partner DJ-producer Ryan Lewis—had taken a years-long break from HIV activism and education when she graced our cover. "It was me coming back to HIV activism after 10 years of not being too involved," Lewis, 60, recalls.

To show gratitude for surviving 30 years with HIV, in 2014, Lewis started the 30/30 Project, aiming to build 30 health care centers around the world to last for at least 30 years. The first to open was in Malawi.

Five years later, Lewis is proud to say that, working alongside respected global aid groups like Partners in Health, she's expecting to fully fund all 30 of her facilities. "It's been very fulfilling, but it's also been a ton of work," she says.

With four grandkids and another on the way, "I'm ready to put some time into my personal life." She laughs at how she imagines the HIV community reacted to her cover appearance.

"It wasn't like, 'Oh, who's this new person?' It was like, 'Oh, she's back.' I'm so excited to not have to be a public person anymore."

For more information and to donate, go to 3030project.org.

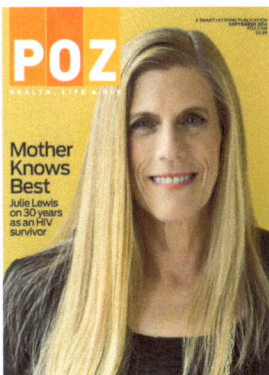

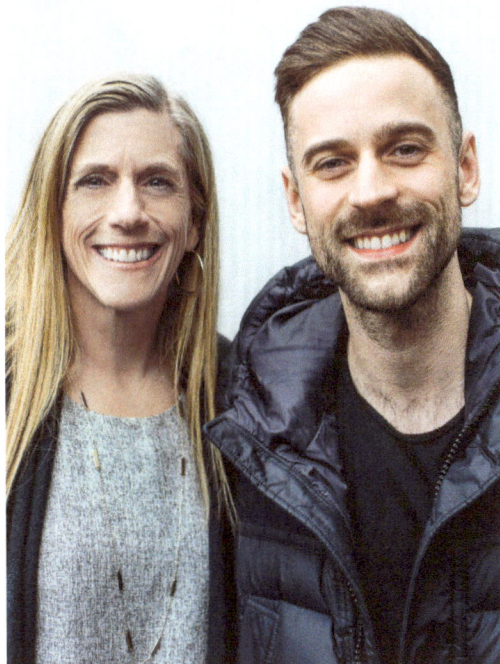

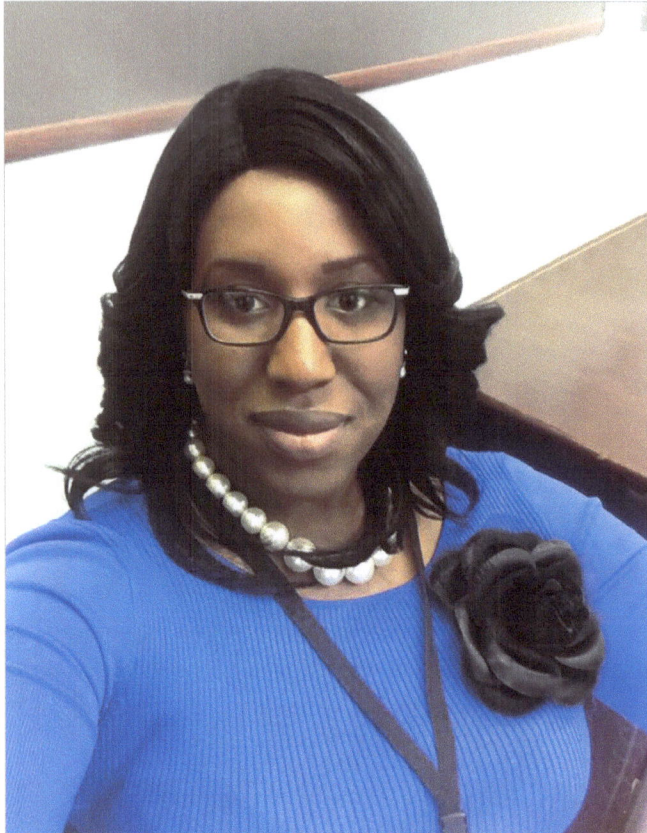

MARCH 2015

Octavia Lewis

"That article opened many doors for me," says Lewis about her 2015 cover story, which details her HIV journey. A lot has changed for her over the past years—she separated from her husband, Shawn Lopez (who also appeared in the article), adopted her foster son, Ethan ("He's now 5!"), and has become one of the nation's leading transgender activists.

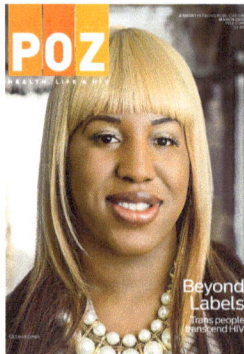

"That article proved so many things that a lot of trans people are told are not possible: a) you can live with HIV; b) you can be a wife; c) you can be a mother; and d) you can be gainfully employed." But having it all was just the beginning.

Now on the board of Positive Women's Network–USA, Lewis is a founding member at Positively Trans and has traveled the world sharing her story. "I'm also still doing stuff locally," she says, donating a lot of her time mentoring trans youth, "just telling them that you can be whoever you choose to be."

JANUARY/FEBRUARY 2016

Ashton P. Woods

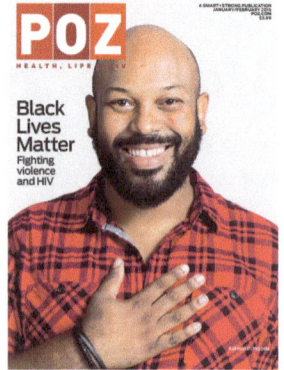

"It wasn't my idea to appear in POZ," says Woods, one of Houston's foremost Black Lives Matter (BLM) activists, when asked about his cover story. "I actually heard through [a friend] that you guys were interested in navigating the BLM movement while HIV positive and Black."

In fact, Woods had a long history as an organizer before gracing the cover of POZ, having started out as an activist in the late '90s after founding one of the first gay-straight alliances in Texas. His aim throughout the years? To ensure that Black people, particularly LGBT Black people, are engaged in politics and viewing their work intersectionally.

Appearing in POZ was perfect. "My reaction when the article came out was the same as everyone else's: How did this happen? Congratulations!" Over the past two years, Woods has continued to organize with BLM and beyond.

He has even filed to run for Houston City Council in 2019. "Election Day is on my birthday," Woods jokes when asked about his future plans for intersectional advocacy.

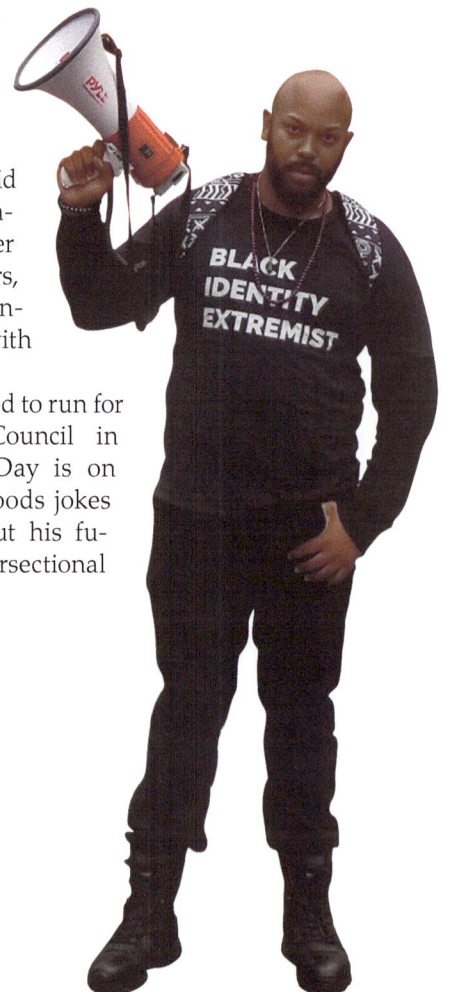

(LEWIS, WOODS, MUÑOZ, TERRY) COURTESY OF INDIVIDUALS

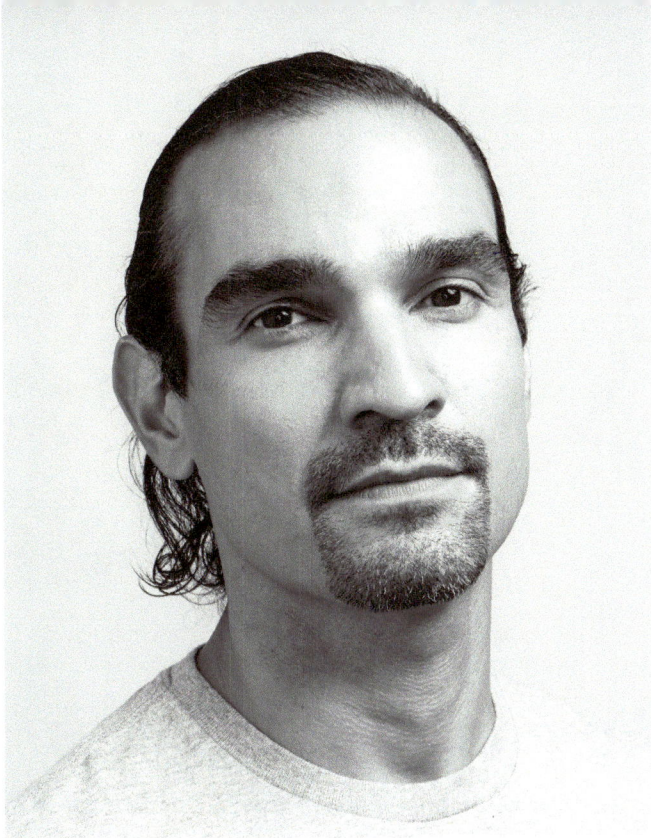

OCTOBER/NOVEMBER 2016

Javier Muñoz

Muñoz was already famous by the time he appeared on POZ's cover, having succeeded his good friend and fellow Puerto Rican New Yorker Lin-Manuel Miranda in the title role of the Broadway blockbuster musical *Hamilton*. In fact, Miranda had bestowed him his own hashtag, #Javilton.

And Muñoz had already made a splash—and been honored by GMHC—for coming out as both a cancer survivor and a person living with HIV in The New York Times right before he stepped into the lead role, saying he wanted newly diagnosed young folks to have the kind of role model he lacked when he was diagnosed in 2002.

Since leaving *Hamilton* in early 2018 after a year-plus run as the lead and finishing up a stint on the TV show *Shadowhunters*, "I've spent time nurturing my relationship with my partner while reconnecting with family and friends," he says. "A show like *Hamilton* takes over your entire life, so this year has been about finding balance with my personal life as well as my professional life."

Muñoz says being on POZ's cover "was an honor and [led to] the greatest show of support I could ever wish for. That energy fed me, and I hope to keep returning that support to others living with HIV or AIDS for as long as I live."

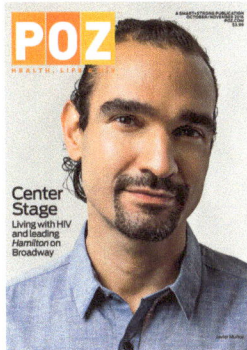

JANUARY/FEBRUARY 2017

Marvell Terry

Terry was one of the folks spotlighted in the cover story, which addressed the structural, social and health barriers that challenge Black gay and bisexual men at the center of the epidemic in the South.

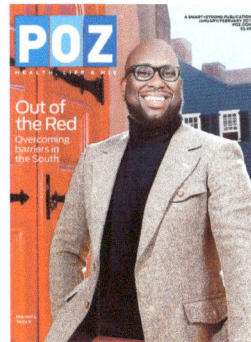

"I was excited and nervous," he says about his decision to speak out in the article.

But the value of the work Terry continues to do on behalf of men who have sex with men in the South is undeniable.

The 33-year-old advocate is the creator of the Red Door Foundation, an HIV advocacy group in his native Memphis, and founder of the annual Saving Ourselves Symposium, a conference by and for Black LGBTQ living in the South that's focused on health, wellness and social justice.

"My advocacy and activism have certainly expanded since I was featured in POZ," he adds. "I now look at HIV at the intersection of so many other issues that impact Black and brown communities, such as homelessness, food deserts and poverty. You see I am Black before you know I am living with HIV or gay—and that reality has fueled me in broadening by coalition building and joining other movements."

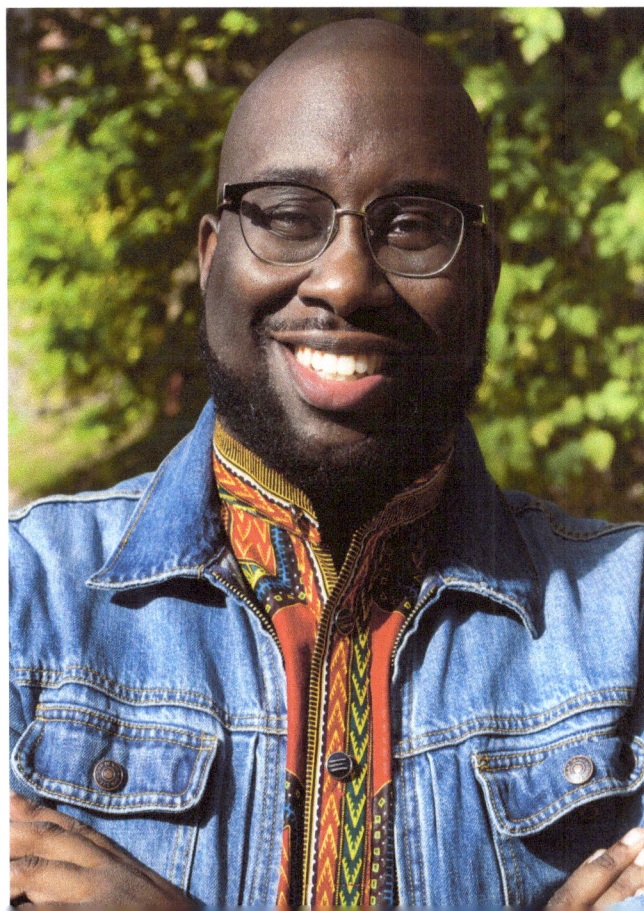

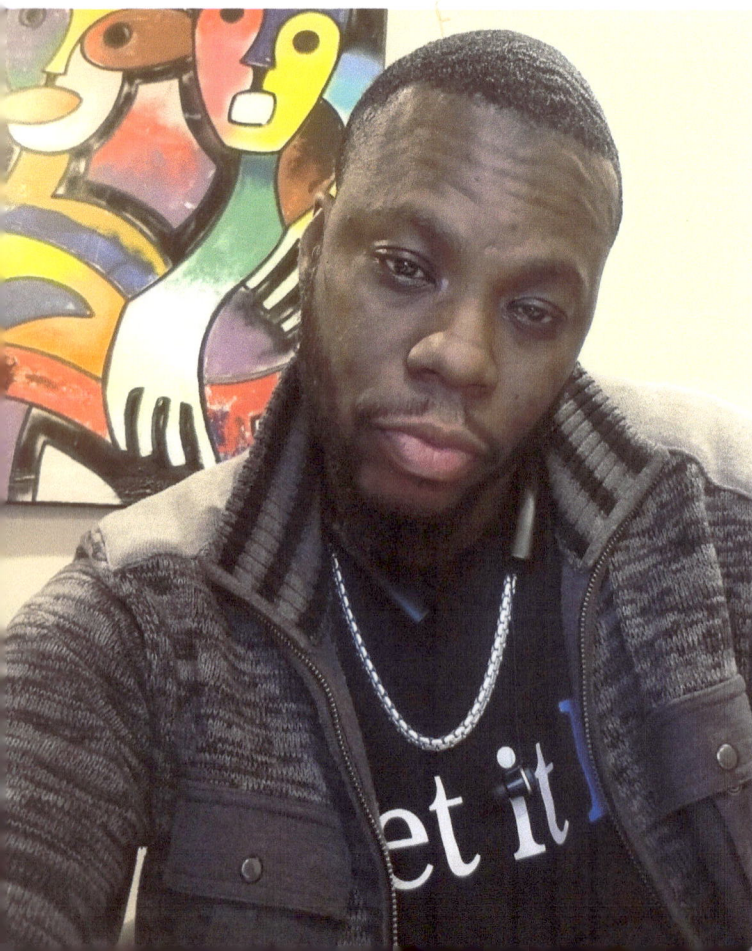

Achim Howard

"I'm just standing up for the trans men who can't stand up for themselves," says Howard when asked about his cover story about fighting erasure and HIV in the transgender community. A few months before the article's publication, he and other trans activists made waves at the United States Conference on AIDS when they stormed the stage to demand better representation at the conference.

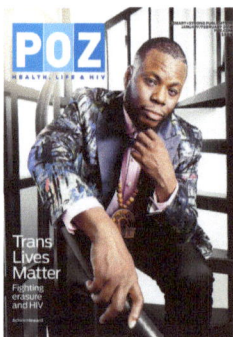

"I remember sitting at a table with all of my sisters at Positively Trans and seeing over and over again that the data for transgender people was just not there. I couldn't take it anymore." More than a year later, Howard is still hard at work in the community, continuing to advocate both as the founder of DC's Trans Men Rising and a Positively Trans board member.

"We are still not being counted. We still need adequate health care. The studies, the data, need to be for us." Because at the end of the day, says Howard, a cover story might be great, but for much of the HIV-positive community, the work has just begun.

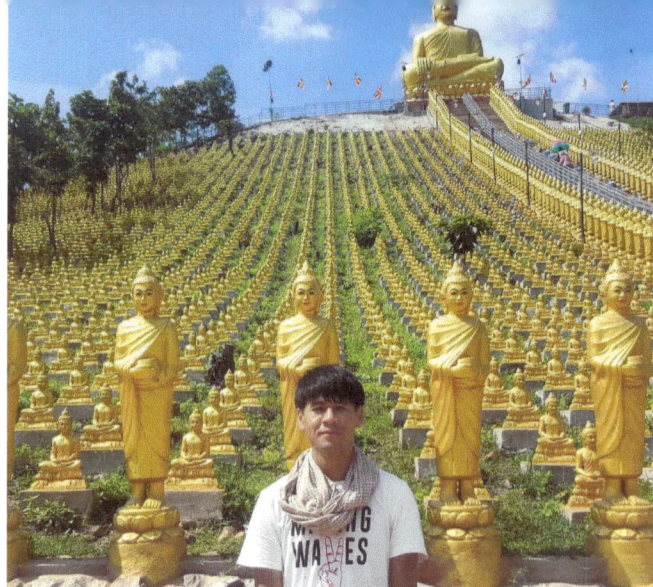

Romany Tin

"I felt proud and empowered knowing that I was fighting for the rights of HIV-positive individuals," says Tin, 24, of his POZ cover.

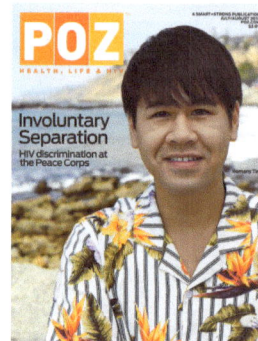

"But at the same time, it frightened me that everyone would know about me and my status. The stigma around it has changed my life, and that is something I would really like to change."

At the time, Tin was in limbo back in the United States after the Peace Corps sent him home from Cambodia, his father's homeland, for testing HIV positive while serving. That move on the part of the agency belied its promise a decade before that it would not dismiss members who test HIV positive and send them home if their treatment and care could be reasonably accommodated (see Jeremiah Johnson on page 78).

Like Johnson, Tin fought the rejection, reaching out not only to Johnson via Treatment Action Group but also to the ACLU and Lambda Legal—all of whom pressed the Peace Corps on why it had to send Tin home from a country with solid access to HIV meds and care. The pushback paid off: The Peace Corps once again said it would no longer send members with HIV home unnecessarily. Tin is back in Cambodia, teaching English.

"I get my treatment and labs here at the hospital in Phnom Penh," he says. "Overall, I'm doing well. Living with HIV hasn't changed much of my habits." Once back in the United States, Tin wants to find decent-paying work, go to grad school for public health and continue working in HIV activism.

His appearance in POZ, he says, "was the first time I felt part of this community. It gave me the confidence to continue my advocacy to fight for people with HIV."

OCTOBER/NOVEMBER 2018

Charles Sanchez

By the time Sanchez made the cover of POZ, he'd been running the blog circuit promoting his now-hit web series, *Merce*—a self-described "sparkly, show tune-y, jazz-handy, middle-aged" extravaganza about what it's like to live with HIV today.

"One of the major impetuses of [starting *Merce*] was that every time I saw a character with HIV on television or in a movie, it was always sad," Sanchez recalls.

Fast-forward to today, and the show—which includes everything from musical interludes about HIV-related diarrhea to heart-wrenching stories about love and acceptance—is in postproduction for its second season, set to debut by fall 2019.

Sanchez can also be found on TheBody.com, where he is currently a contributing editor, as well as at various HIV-related events like AIDSWatch and the United States Conference on AIDS.

"That cover story really validated our project," says Sanchez. "It introduced us to the HIV community in a lovely way so that when I started doing more writing and other kinds of advocacy work, people knew who I was and listened to what I had to say."

(SANCHEZ) BILL WADMAN

ON THE COVER

CREDITS: (1) Jeremy Charles, (2) Euclides Santiago, (3) Meredith Parmelee, (4, 45) Scott Pasfield, (5, 35) Dean Kaufman, (6, 28, 49) Blake Little, (7) Dirk Lindner, (8) Andrew McLeod, (9) Eric Rhein, (10, 12, 19, 26, 27, 30, 36, 37, 55, 62, 63, 69) Bill Wadman, (11) Robin Holland, (13) Ken Probst, (14) Naomi Harris, (15, 18, 46) Jonathan Timmes, (16) Clay Patrick McBride, (17) Scott Morgan, (20) Kristina Marie Krug, (21) Todd Selby, (22) Dean Williams, (23) Kyle Froman, (24) Ryan Ketterman, (25, 58) Jeff Singer, (29) Bryan Regan, (31) Peter James Zielinski/BC/EFA, (32) Troy Plota, (33, 52) Carolyn Jones, (34, 44, 50, 71) Toky, (38) Ben Watts, (39) Ethan Hill, (40) Andrew Melick, (41) Brian Smith, (42, 60) Greg Gorman, (43) Rafa Alvaraez, (47) Joan L. Brown, (48) Jacop Kepler, (51) Toby Burditt, (53) Dean Macadam, (54) Ronnie Arden, (56) Steve Morrison, (57) Roy Inman, (59) Justin Tsucalas, (61) Roddy McDowall, (64) Chris Corrie, (65) Jensen Larson, (66) Frederic Brown/ Agence France-Presse, (67) Ann Marsden, (68) Angel Valentín, (70) Kevin Steele

View this guide on POZ.com for links to all the cover articles.

#		#		#		#		#		#	
1.	Shana Cozad	13.	Pedro Zamora	24.	Charles Tripp	32.	Sean Sasser	47.	Sean Strub	61.	Elizabeth Taylor
2.	Moisés Agosto-Rosario	14.	John Muhammad	25.	Rob Newells	33.	Kiyoshi Kuromiya	48.	Hydeia Broadbent	62.	Tim Murphy
3.	Dog in wig	15.	Linda Scruggs	26.	Fred Hersch	34.	Jeffrey Jenest	49.	Greg Louganis	63.	Rep. Barbara Lee
4.	Bob Bowers		Nathaniel Scruggs	27.	Robert Chodo	35.	Peter Staley	50.	Sherri Lewis	64.	Kory Montoya
5.	Shane Theriot	16.	Stacey Latimer		Campbell	36.	Charles King	51.	Vicki Derdivanis	65.	Reginald T. Brown
6.	Tony Valenzuela	17.	Joseph Sonnabend	28.	Mondo Guerra	37.	Antonio Muñoz	52.	Lisa Tiger		Wanda Brendle-Moss
7.	Andy Bell	18.	Shawn Decker	29.	Janet Kitchen	38.	Stephen Gendin	53.	Kami the Muppet	66.	Song Pengfei
8.	Larry Bryant		Gwenn Barringer		Pat Kelly	39.	Larry Kramer	54.	Mila Vreeland	67.	Emily Carter
9.	*Life Altering Spencer*	19.	Luz de Jesus Roman		Lepena Powell-Reid	40.	Thom Collins		Memory Amya Hunte	68.	L'Orangelis Thomas
10.	Jay W. Walker	20.	Alee Meredith		Juanita Williams	41.	Jesus Sanchez	55.	Nancy Duncan		Negrón
11.	Anthony Salandra		Mitchell Meredith		Margot Kirkland-Isaac	42.	Mary Fisher	56.	Lafayette Sanders	69.	Whitney Joiner
	Marsha Burnett		Yonas Meredith		Vanessa Johnson	43.	Adonis Porch	57.	Jane Fowler		Alysia Abbott
	Ruben Rodriguez	21.	Chloe Dzubilo		Stephanie Laster	44.	Jamar Rogers	58.	Giuliani Alvarenga	70.	Jason Villalobos
12.	Kim Hunter	22.	Michael Jeter	30.	Eileen Mitzman	45.	Marvelyn Brown	59.	Anna Fowlkes	71.	Jake Glaser
	Cesar Carrasco	23.	Salim "Slam" Gauwloos		(Marni Mitzman)	46.	Barb Cardell		Paul Johns	72.	U=U
	Perry Halkitis		Carlton Wilborn	31.	Broadway Cares dancers		Sharon DeCuir	60.	Brian Grillo		

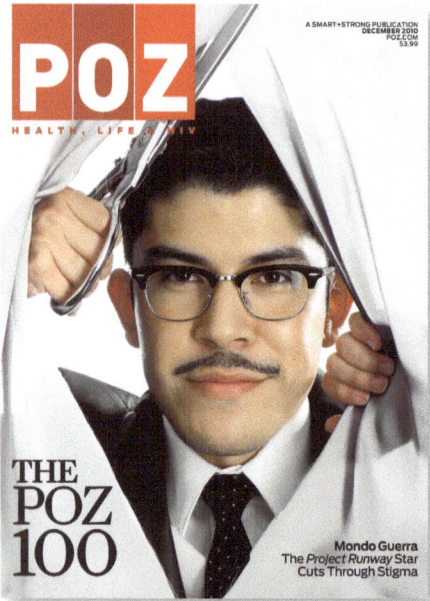

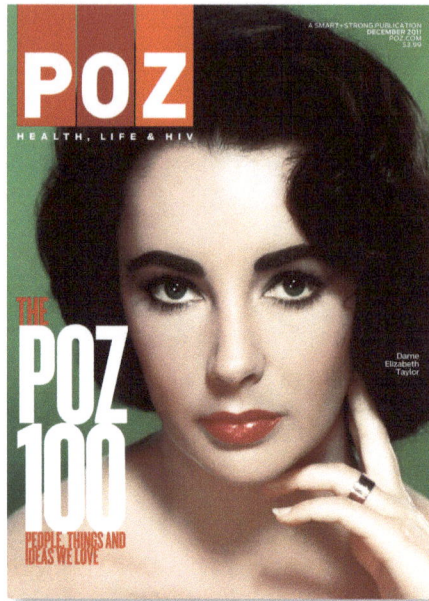

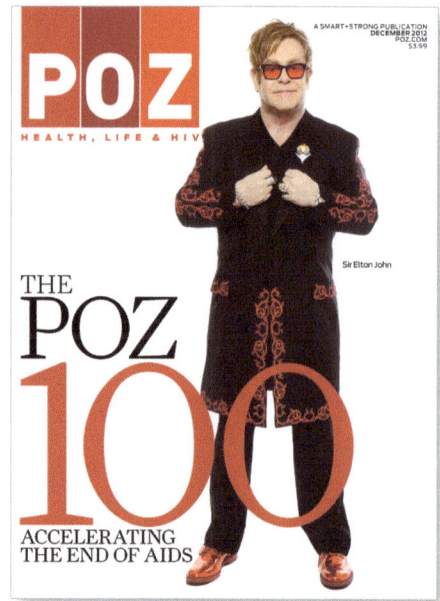

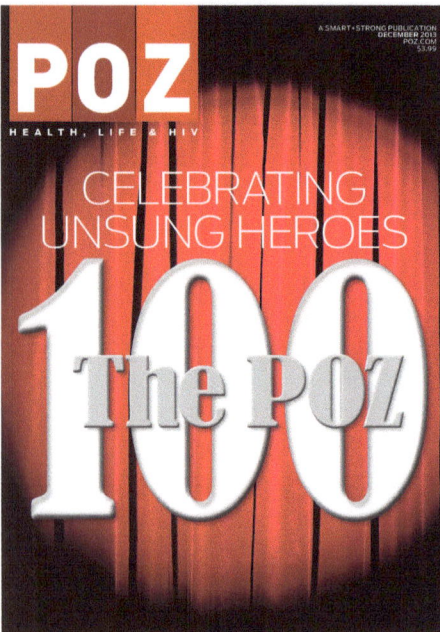

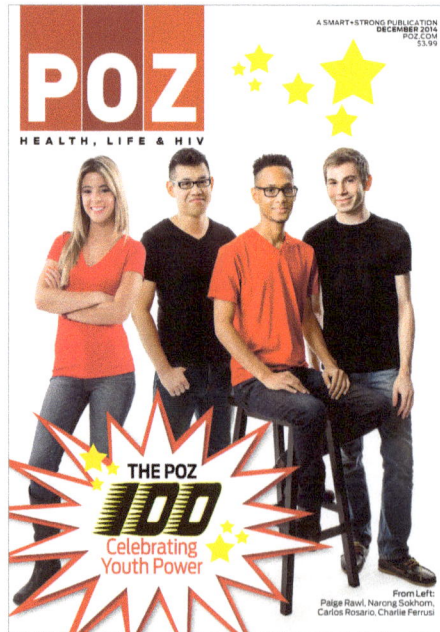

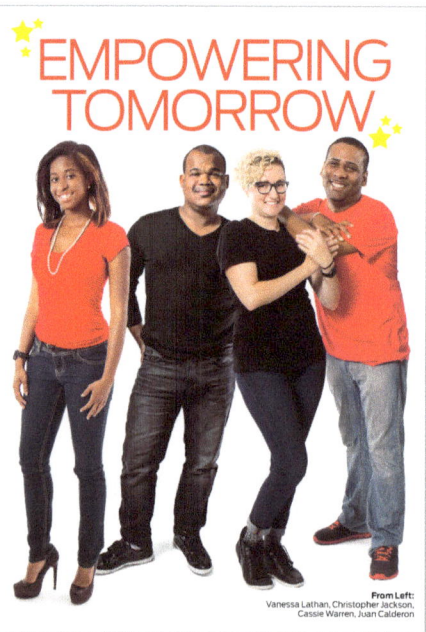

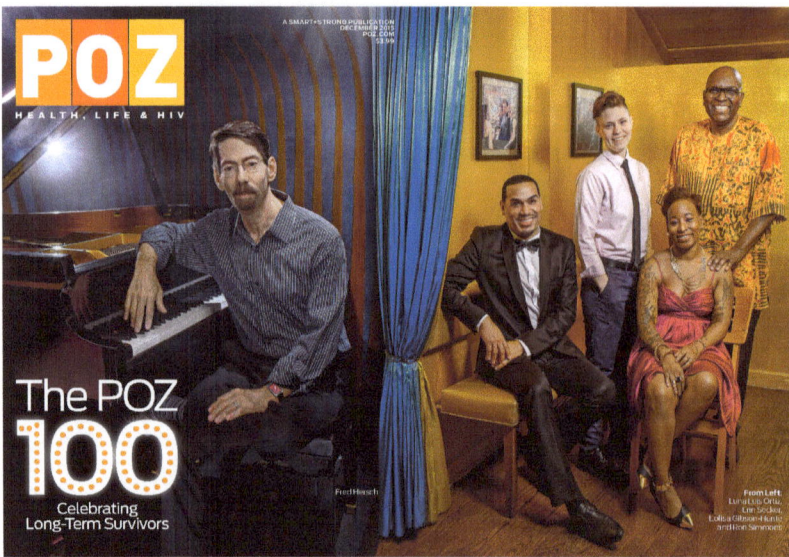

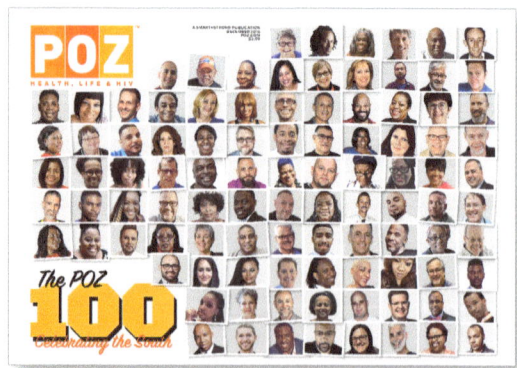

Covers of December issues featuring the POZ 100 list. This page, top: 2010, 2011, 2012; middle: 2013, 2014; bottom: 2015, 2016. Right page, top: 2017; bottom: 2018.

The POZ 100

MUCH HAS CHANGED SINCE OUR ANNUAL LIST honoring HIV/AIDS advocates debuted in 2010. There's still a lot of work to be done to end the epidemic, but the years since we published our first list have seen the creation of the first National HIV/AIDS Strategy and the lifting of the HIV travel ban, which led to the return of the International AIDS Conference to the United States. There have also been a number of significant scientific breakthroughs.

For example, we now have pre-exposure prophylaxis (PrEP) to prevent HIV, and we know that treatment for the virus equals prevention when people living with HIV can maintain an undetectable viral load.

A decade ago, the Obama administration gave HIV advocates hope for a renewed effort against the virus at the federal level. It was in this context that the first POZ 100 list was born. We spotlighted 100 warriors in the fight against AIDS in order to support their work. We wanted to honor their service and inspire them to carry on. Today, that inspiration and support is needed more than ever.

The list has a different focus each year, such as youth, women or long-term survivors. It also varies from including only people living with HIV to sometimes including HIV-negative allies. Despite those differences, the goal remains the same—to honor those in the HIV/AIDS struggle for their work.

POZ has always been a mirror for the community, so we wanted to reflect all the efforts being made by so many. While some honorees have been well known, many of them were known only to their local communities before they were nationally recognized. No list is ever definitive, but we've done our best to make each POZ 100 list representative of the epidemic.

We celebrate the achievements of all our POZ 100 honorees!

Visit poz.com/page/poz-100 for more information.

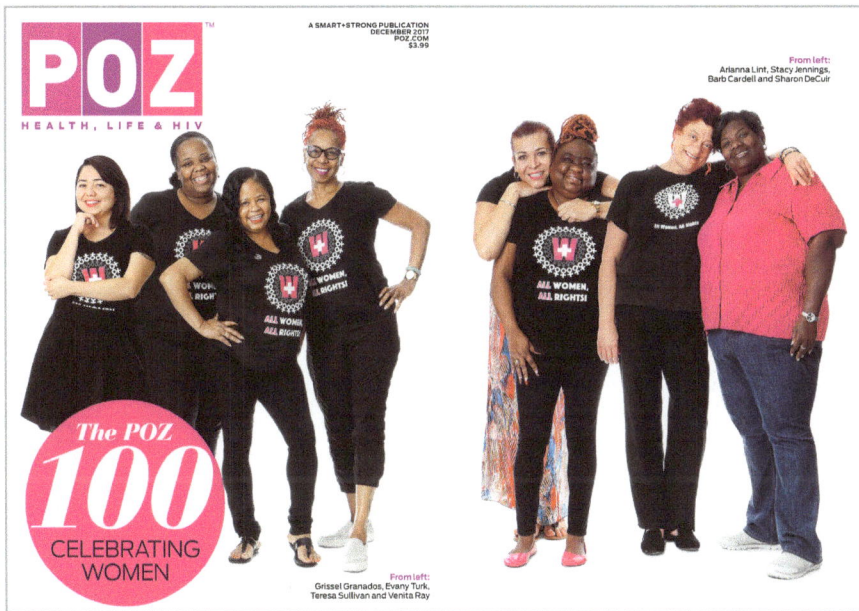

POZ
HEALTH, LIFE & HIV

A SMART+STRONG PUBLICATION
DECEMBER 2017
POZ.COM
$3.99

From left:
Arianna Lint, Stacy Jennings,
Barb Cardell and Sharon DeCuir

The POZ
100
CELEBRATING
WOMEN

From left:
Grissel Granados, Evany Turk,
Teresa Sullivan and Venita Ray

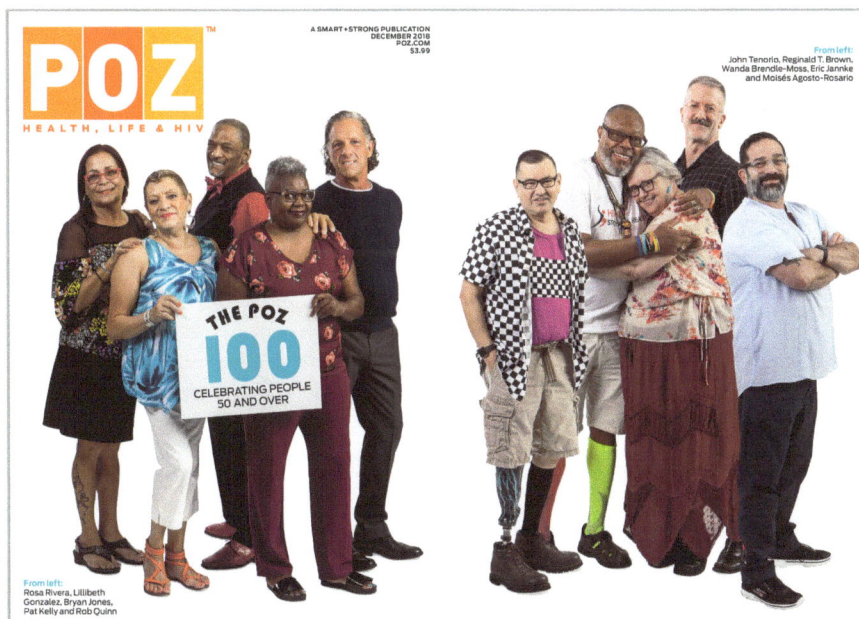

POZ
HEALTH, LIFE & HIV

A SMART+STRONG PUBLICATION
DECEMBER 2018
POZ.COM
$3.99

From left:
John Tenorio, Reginald T. Brown,
Wanda Brendle-Moss, Eric Jannke
and Moisés Agosto-Rosario

THE POZ
100
CELEBRATING PEOPLE
50 AND OVER

From left:
Rosa Rivera, Lillibeth
Gonzalez, Bryan Jones,
Pat Kelly and Rob Quinn

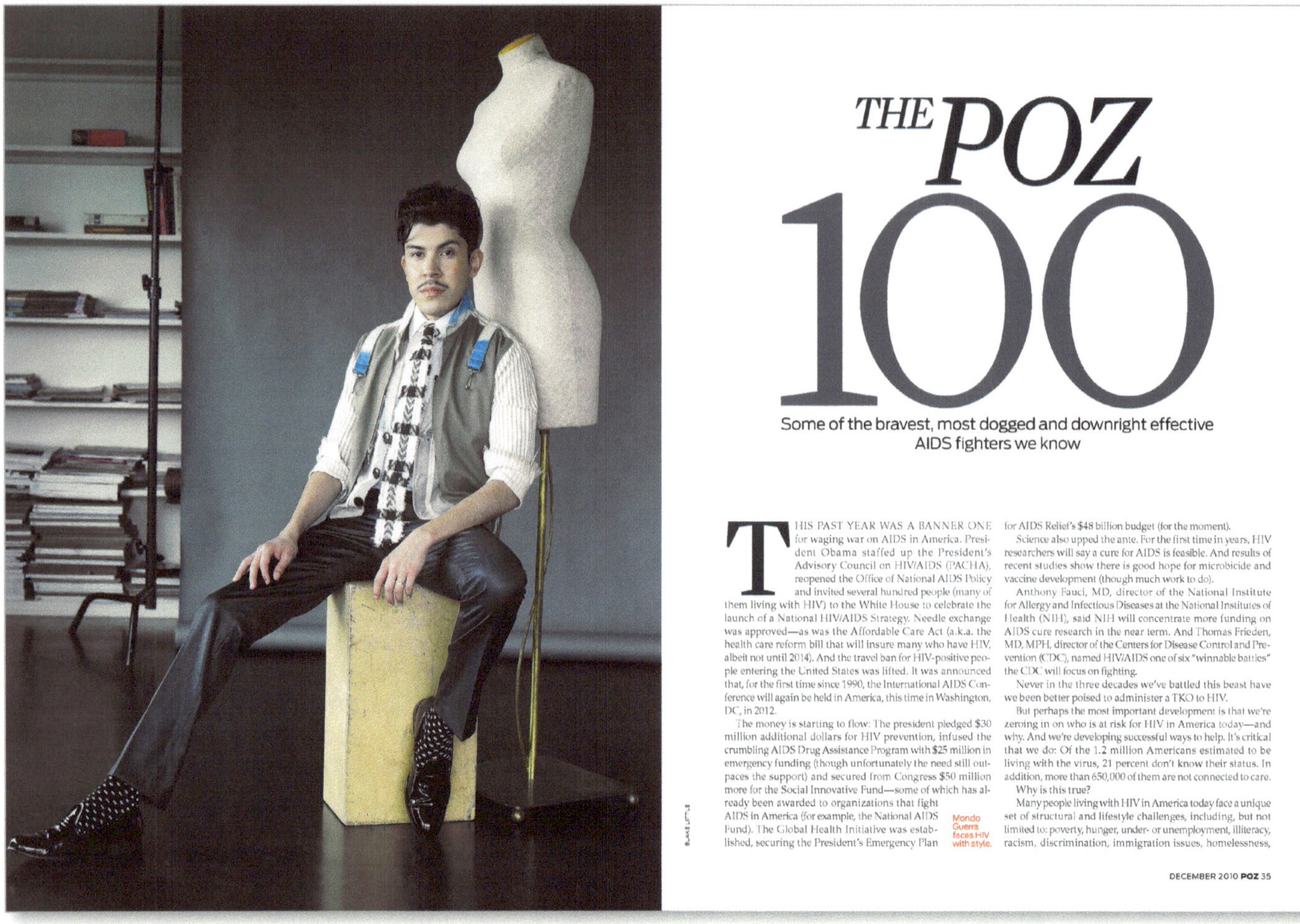

THE POZ 100

Some of the bravest, most dogged and downright effective AIDS fighters we know

THIS PAST YEAR WAS A BANNER ONE for waging war on AIDS in America. President Obama staffed up the President's Advisory Council on HIV/AIDS (PACHA), reopened the Office of National AIDS Policy and invited several hundred people (many of them living with HIV) to the White House to celebrate the launch of a National HIV/AIDS Strategy. Needle exchange was approved—as was the Affordable Care Act (a.k.a. the health care reform bill that will insure many who have HIV, albeit not until 2014). And the travel ban for HIV-positive people entering the United States was lifted. It was announced that, for the first time since 1990, the International AIDS Conference will again be held in America, this time in Washington, DC, in 2012.

The money is starting to flow: The president pledged $30 million additional dollars for HIV prevention, infused the crumbling AIDS Drug Assistance Program with $25 million in emergency funding (though unfortunately the need still outpaces the support) and secured from Congress $50 million more for the Social Innovative Fund—some of which has already been awarded to organizations that fight AIDS in America (for example, the National AIDS Fund). The Global Health Initiative was established, securing the President's Emergency Plan for AIDS Relief's $48 billion budget (for the moment).

Mondo Guerra faces HIV with style.

Science also upped the ante. For the first time in years, HIV researchers will say a cure for AIDS is feasible. And results of recent studies show there is good hope for microbicide and vaccine development (though much work to do).

Anthony Fauci, MD, director of the National Institute for Allergy and Infectious Diseases at the National Institutes of Health (NIH), said NIH will concentrate more funding on AIDS cure research in the near term. And Thomas Frieden, MD, MPH, director of the Centers for Disease Control and Prevention (CDC), named HIV/AIDS one of six "winnable battles" the CDC will focus on fighting.

Never in the three decades we've battled this beast have we been better poised to administer a TKO to HIV.

But perhaps the most important development is that we're zeroing in on who is at risk for HIV in America today—and why. And we're developing successful ways to help. It's critical that we do: Of the 1.2 million Americans estimated to be living with the virus, 21 percent don't know their status. In addition, more than 650,000 of them are not connected to care.

Why is this true?

Many people living with HIV in America today face a unique set of structural and lifestyle challenges, including, but not limited to: poverty, hunger, under- or unemployment, illiteracy, racism, discrimination, immigration issues, homelessness,

DECEMBER 2010 POZ 35

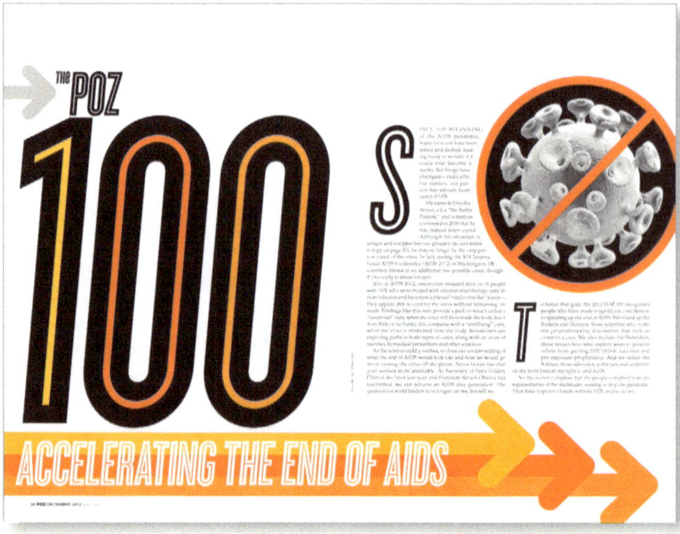

Each year the POZ 100 list focuses on a specific group of honorees, sometimes honoring people living with HIV and other times including HIV-negative allies—2010: AIDS fighters; 2011: people, things and ideas we love; 2012: accelerating the end of AIDS; 2013: unsung heroes; 2014: youth; 2015: long-term survivors; 2016: advocates from the South; 2017: women; 2018: people 50 and over. The 2019 list will honor trans advocates.

The features section of each December issue is dedicated to the POZ 100 list and includes descriptions of the honorees. Here are spreads of POZ 100 lists introducing past honorees and detailing the criteria for inclusion on that year's list. Left page, top: 2010; bottom: 2011, 2012. Right page, top: 2013, 2014; middle: 2015, 2016; bottom: 2017, 2018.

2010

April/May

COVER: Miss Universe Stefanía Fernández discusses global advocacy with Aid for AIDS executive director Jesús Aguais (**3**). **INSIDE:** Mark Harrington and the team behind the Treatment Action Group; meet one of the first people to enter the United States after the lifting of the 22-year ban on travelers living with HIV. **PLUS:** Miss America Caressa Cameron on why she uses her platform to fight HIV.

Adoption Issues

January/February

COVER: Phill Wilson and the Black AIDS Institute launch the new national campaign "Greater Than AIDS." **INSIDE:** How one HIV-positive man fought back to adopt a child (**1**); Jane Aronson helps kids across the globe via the Worldwide Orphans Foundation. **PLUS:** Fitness coach Valerie Wojciechowicz offers small steps for success.

June

COVER: Tim Horn—with his boxers Buster and Lucy—shares how our pets can make us healthier (**4**). **INSIDE:** What the newly signed Patient Protection and Affordable Care Act of 2010 means for you; Gym Class Heroes front man Travis McCoy promotes HIV prevention to young people. **PLUS:** Marvelyn Brown's activism lands her image on the back of Doritos bags across the country.

March

COVER: Vicki Derdivanis—and six other wonder women—share how to live with HIV and help other sisters along the way (**2**). **INSIDE:** The need to know more about how HIV affects menstruation and menopause; long-time advocates Dawn Averitt Bridge and Mary Fisher discuss why women are particularly vulnerable to the virus. **PLUS:** U.S. Senator Kirsten Gillibrand on why she's involved in HIV advocacy.

July/August

COVER: The global AIDS crisis needs our attention—and funding. **INSIDE:** How Consolee Nishimwe survived the Rwandan genocide and is surviving with HIV (**5**); dealing with the deadly aftermath of the earthquake in Haiti. **PLUS:** Some strategies for dealing with chronic pain.

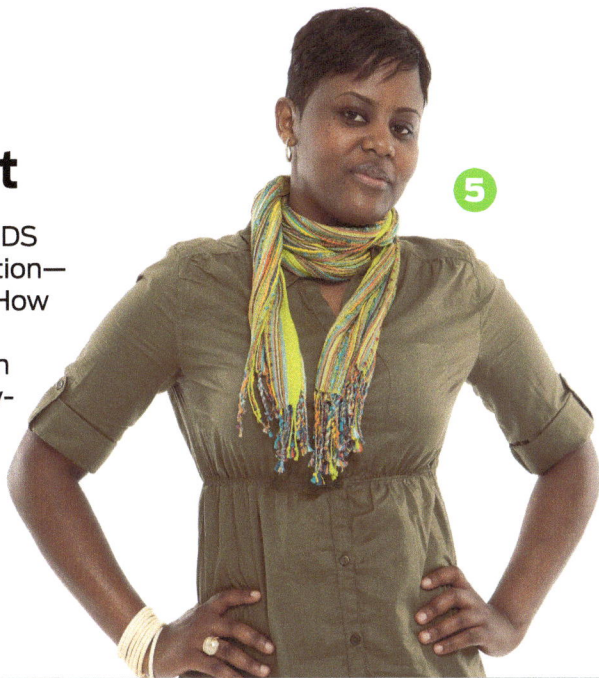

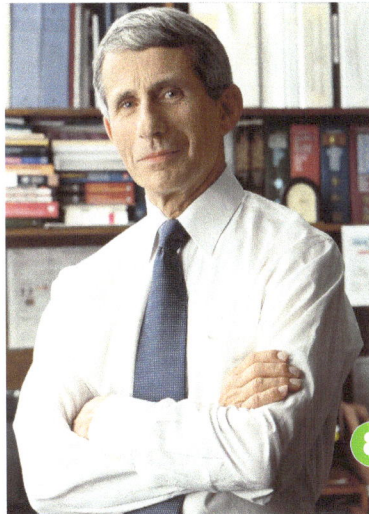

October/November

COVER: A look at the current state of cure research and what we need to do next. **INSIDE:** Jeff Crowley on the release and implementation of the National HIV/AIDS Strategy; Anthony Fauci, MD, on finding a cure and working with the HIV community (**8**). **PLUS:** The People Living With HIV Stigma Index documents people's experiences with HIV stigma and discrimination in more than 20 countries.

September

COVER: The ex-gay movement uses HIV as a scare tactic and puts everyone at a higher risk for the virus (**6**). **INSIDE:** Medical marijuana helps some people living with HIV; the importance of remembering Ryan White (**7**). **PLUS:** Steve Morrison's haunting portraits from the early days of the epidemic.

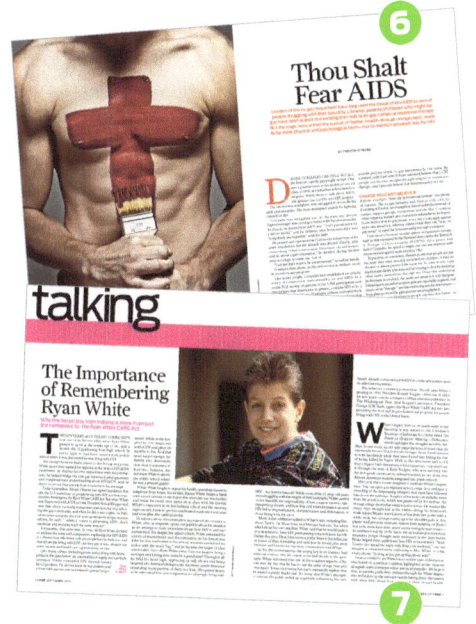

Thou Shalt Fear AIDS

The Importance of Remembering Ryan White

December

COVER: POZ pays tribute to *Project Runway* star Mondo Guerra and 99 other HIV advocates in the first annual POZ 100 (**9**). **INSIDE:** The documentary *Bad Blood* chronicles how the hemophilia community fought to protect the world's blood supply from HIV; Bill T. Jones and Jerry Herman are 2010 Kennedy Center honorees; Pepsi offers a refreshing way to combat HIV. **PLUS:** Jacki Gethner uses her healing touch to improve the lives of people living with HIV.

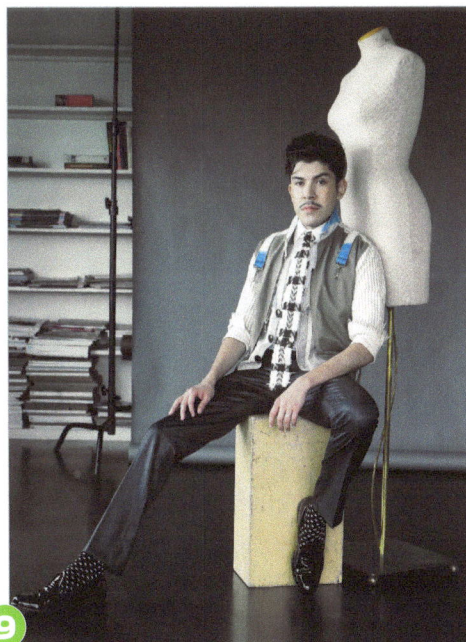

THE POZ 100

Some of the bravest, most dogged and downright effective AIDS fighters we know

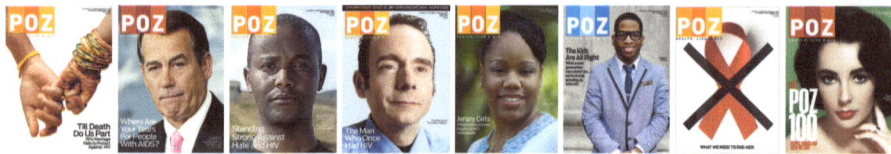

THE YEAR IN POZ

2011

January/February

COVER: In certain societies, marriage can be a barrier to preventing HIV. **INSIDE:** Eric Sawyer, a cofounder of ACT UP and Housing Works, reflects on 30 years of survival with HIV (1); the POZ Safer Sex-O-Meter. **PLUS:** Stigma and discrimination ignite the flames of the HIV epidemic in Southern states (2).

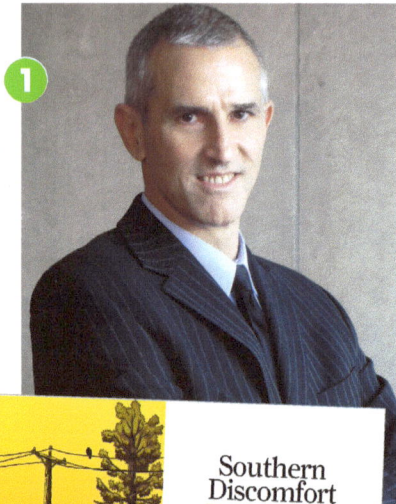

March

COVER: Speaker John Boehner and other House Republicans vow to reverse President Barack Obama's health care initiatives. **INSIDE:** Taming bad hair and HIV is all in a day's work; discovering the keys to HIV non-progressors (3). **PLUS:** A new phone app helps you locate nearby free condoms.

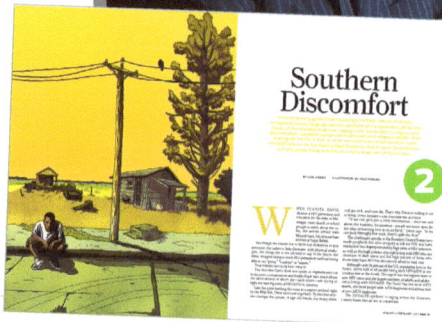

April/May

COVER: David Kuria risks his life every day in Kenya advocating for the rights of LGBT people in Africa and around the world. **INSIDE:** Seven tips for receiving your mail-order meds on time. **PLUS:** Elton Naswood provides HIV education to Native American gay men in Los Angeles (4).

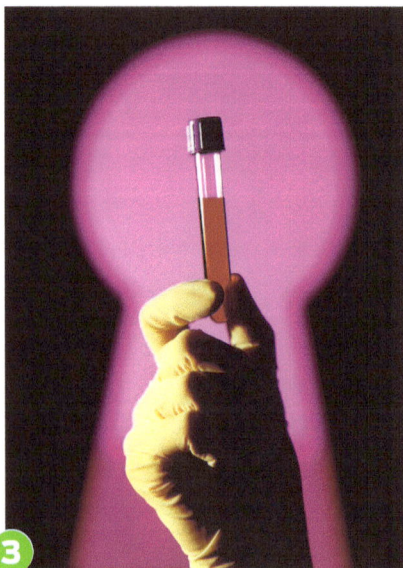

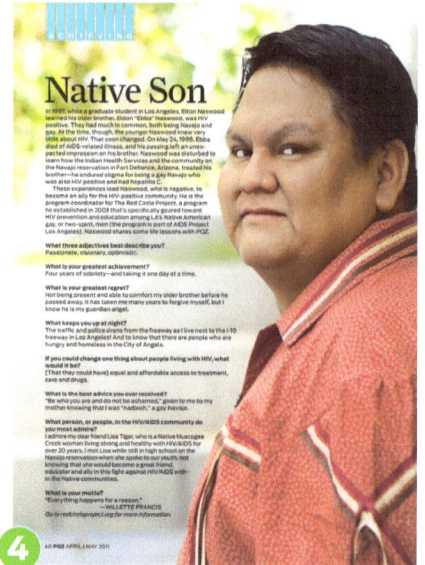

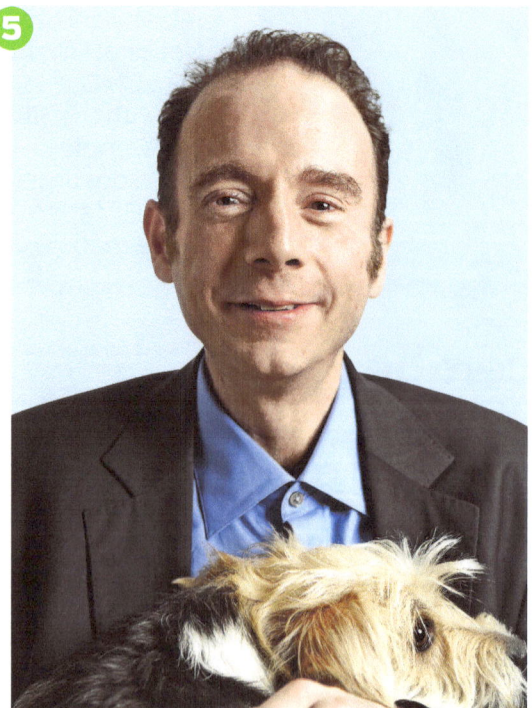

June

COVER: Timothy Ray Brown, also known as "the Berlin Patient," is the first man to be declared cured of HIV (5). **INSIDE:** Michael Gottlieb, MD, the doctor who diagnosed the first AIDS cases, reflects on 30 years of the epidemic. **PLUS:** Remembering long-time AIDS activist Dame Elizabeth Taylor.

July/August

COVER: Dottie Rains shares her story to shed light on the high rates of HIV among women of color living in New Jersey. **INSIDE:** The HPTN 052 study confirms that taking antiretroviral meds and maintaining an undetectable viral load reduces the risk of transmitting the virus to a sexual partner by 96% among heterosexual couples; *The Normal Heart* goes to Broadway (6). **PLUS:** Barbara Joseph provides HIV education through Positive Efforts (7).

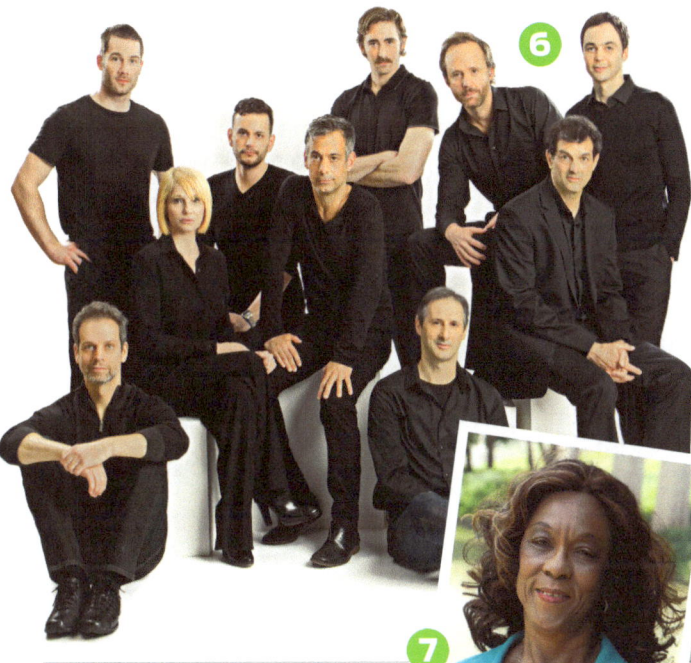

September

COVER: Lafayette Sanders and others of his generation talk about sex, survival and what it's like growing up with HIV (8). **INSIDE:** A portion of the funds raised from an auction of Elizabeth Taylor's jewels will benefit her eponymous AIDS foundation. **PLUS:** When he's not running a marathon to raise money for AIDS, David Munar keeps the AIDS Foundation of Chicago running smoothly.

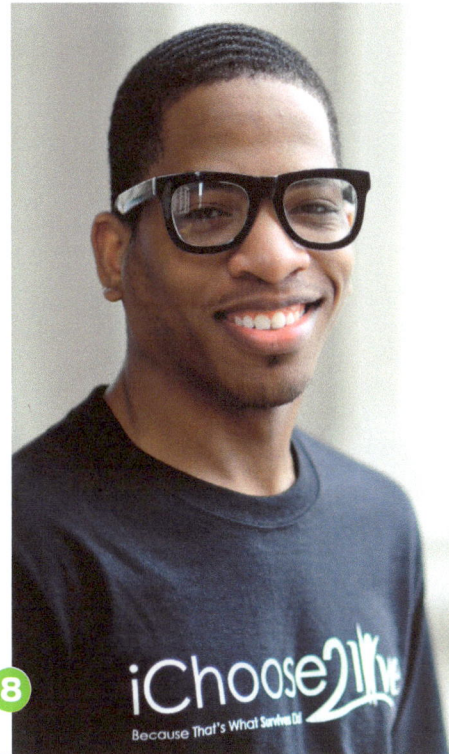

December

COVER: This year's POZ 100 celebrates the people, things and ideas reinventing and improving how we wipe out HIV. **INSIDE:** Protecting the brain from HIV; the bipartisan Congressional HIV/AIDS Caucus is launched to fight the virus. **PLUS:** Dionne Warwick talks about the early days of the epidemic and why she's still fighting for the cause (10).

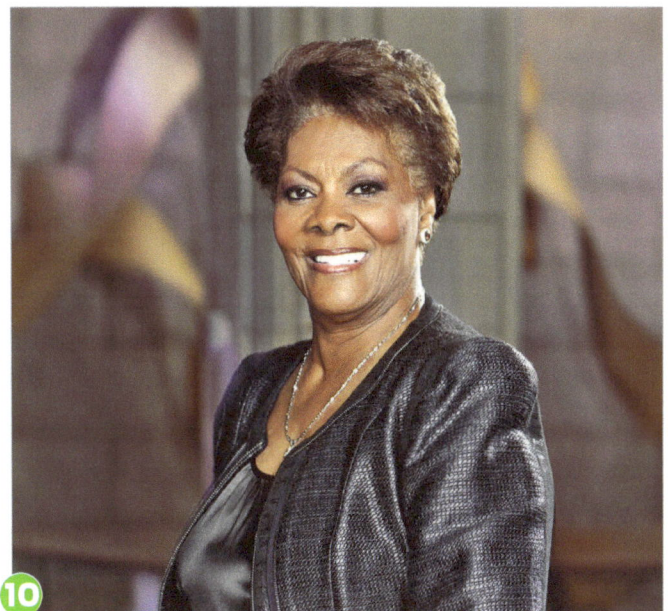

October/November

COVER: Our suggestions for the key things we must do to rid the world of AIDS (9). **INSIDE:** The CDC's Kevin Fenton on a new approach to prevent HIV in the communities most at risk; the debate about pre-exposure prophylaxis, or PrEP, heats up over the summer. **PLUS:** A peek into the HIV pipeline.

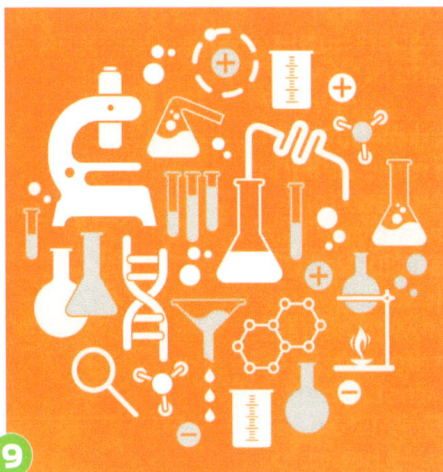

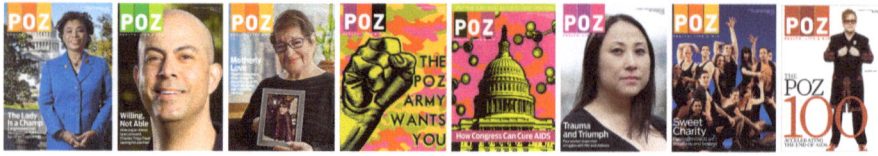

THE YEAR IN POZ

2012

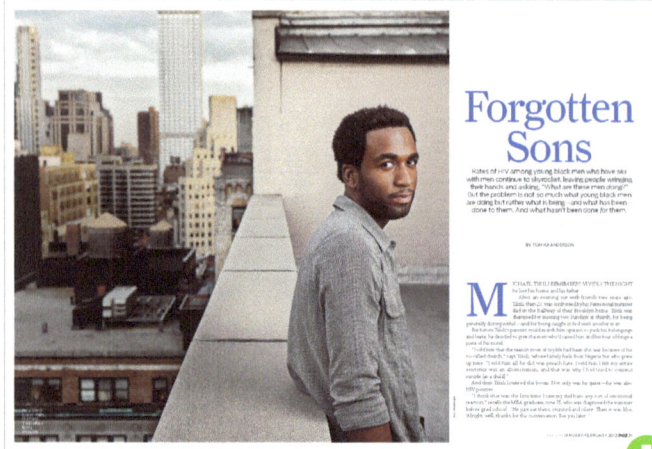

Forgotten Sons

Rates of HIV among young black men who have sex with men continue to skyrocket, leaving people wringing their hands and asking, "What are these men doing?" But the problem is not so much what young black men are doing but rather what is being—and what has been—done to them. And what hasn't been done for them.

BY TOM HUMAN SOMETHING

M ICHAEL TIKILI REMEMBERS VIVIDLY THE NIGHT he lost his home and his father.

January/February

COVER: Congresswoman Barbara Lee fearlessly leads the charge on Capitol Hill for people with HIV.
INSIDE: HIV is just one symptom of the larger issues affecting Michael Tikili and other young Black men who have sex with men (**1**); where you live in the United States influences how well you live with the virus. **PLUS:** How to keep your heart healthy.

March

COVER: Charles Tripp can't donate a portion of his liver to save his partner because federal law forbids people living with HIV from being organ donors. **INSIDE:** Photographer and filmmaker James Houston talks about his latest project, a movie about teenage sexual health titled *Let's Talk About Sex*; Americans are growing old with HIV. **PLUS:** A toy-sized terrier raises money for AIDS (**2**).

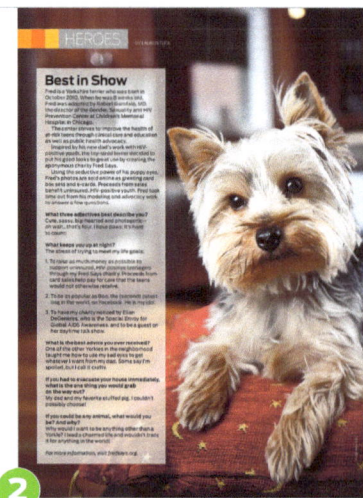

HEROES

Best in Show

April/May

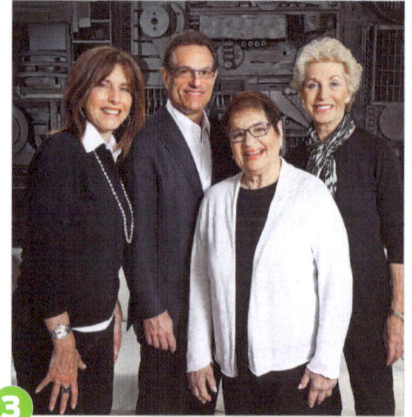

COVER: Eileen Mitzman continues to fight for people with HIV even after losing her daughter to AIDS two decades ago (**3**). **INSIDE:** Meet the warriors working to get more people on treatment in order to slow the spread of HIV; David France hopes his documentary *How to Survive a Plague* will inspire the next generation of HIV activists. **PLUS:** Products to help you relax and rejuvenate.

June

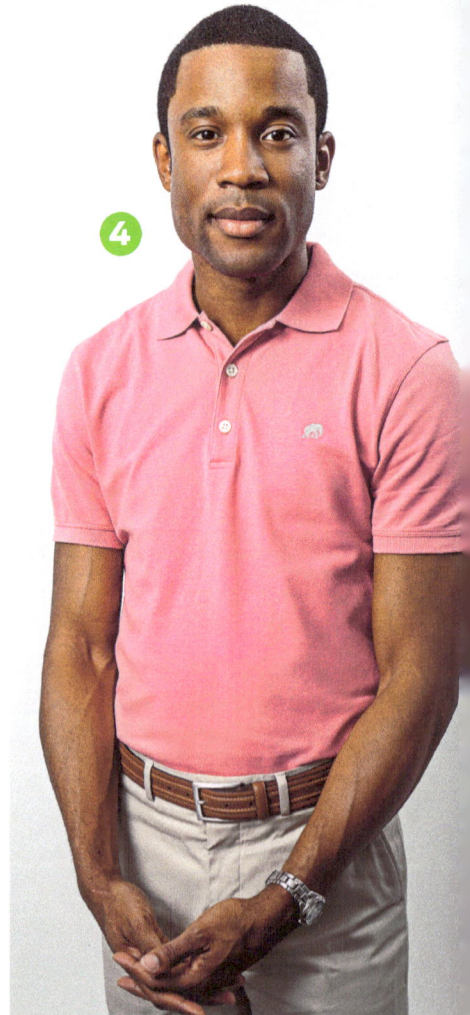

COVER: Editor-in-chief Regan Hofmann summons readers to serve in the POZ Army to advocate for the end of AIDS in anticipation of the International AIDS Conference in Washington, DC. **INSIDE:** Robert Suttle and others share their HIV criminalization stories and their crusade for health, welfare and justice (**4**); teaching women how to navigate safer sex. **PLUS:** Artist Avram Finkelstein uses his art to inspire activism and highlight injustice.

July/August

COVER: In preparation for the 2012 International AIDS Conference, POZ offers Congress a seven-item must-do list—including tackling homophobia and racism, decriminalizing HIV, encouraging safer drug use—if we are to end AIDS in our lifetime (5). **INSIDE:** A new film explores why the American South has not succeeded in its struggle to break free of AIDS; Françoise Barré-Sinoussi, co-discoverer of HIV, discusses the hunt for a cure (6). **PLUS:** Magic Johnson has a new Medicaid plan for Florida.

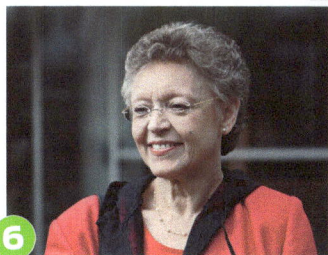

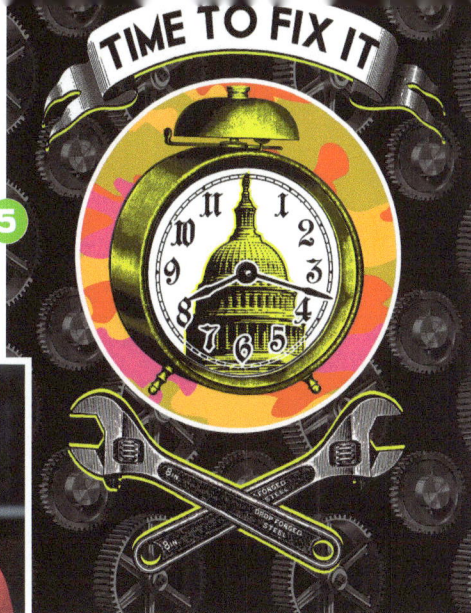

September

COVER: Cecilia Chung has struggled with violence and HIV. In our feature, Valerie Holmes and Kat Griffith also share how they've dealt with HIV-related trauma (7). **INSIDE:** Jim Hubbard on his documentary, *United in Anger: A History of ACT UP*; an HIV campaign inspired by *Fifty Shades of Grey*. **PLUS:** Readers weigh in on the first at-home rapid HIV test.

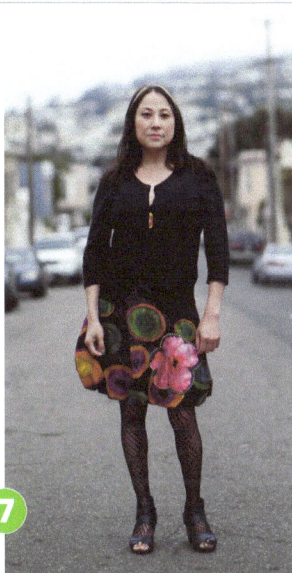

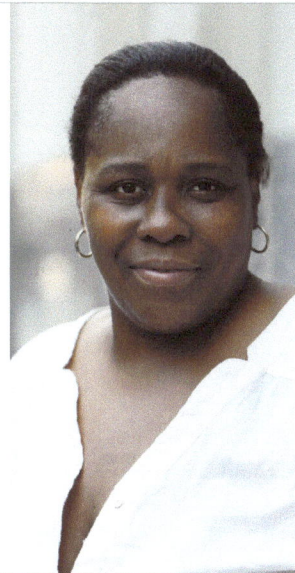

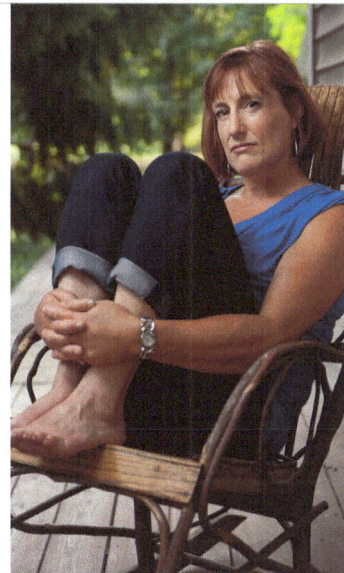

October/November

COVER: Broadway Cares/Equity Fights AIDS supports HIV and family service programs nationwide as well as AIDS research and advocacy. **INSIDE:** Scott A. Schoettes of Lambda Legal outlines the battle being waged in U.S. courts over HIV criminalization; highlights from the 19th International AIDS Conference in Washington, DC (8). **PLUS:** David Heckerman, the guy who invented Microsoft's email spam filter, is now fighting another type of invader: HIV.

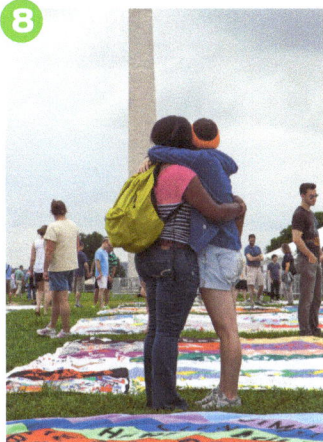

December

COVER: Sir Elton John is one of 100 people recognized in the 2012 POZ 100 for helping to speed up the end of AIDS (9). **INSIDE:** An excerpt from John's new book, *Love Is the Cure*, reveals that he wishes he had done more to fight AIDS during the early days of the epidemic; an iPad video game hopes to teach HIV prevention skills. **PLUS:** Over-the-counter HIV tests: helpful or harmful?

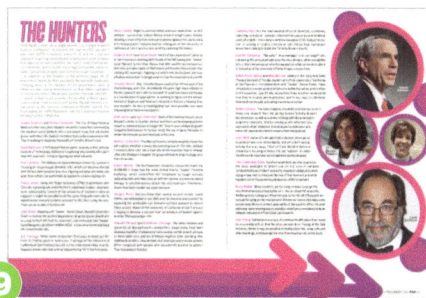

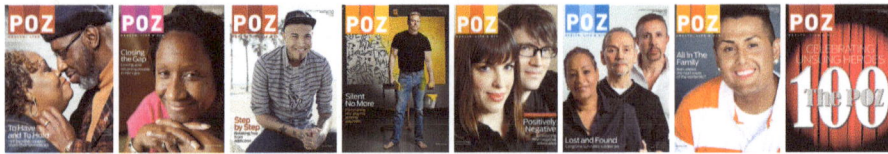

THE YEAR IN POZ

2013

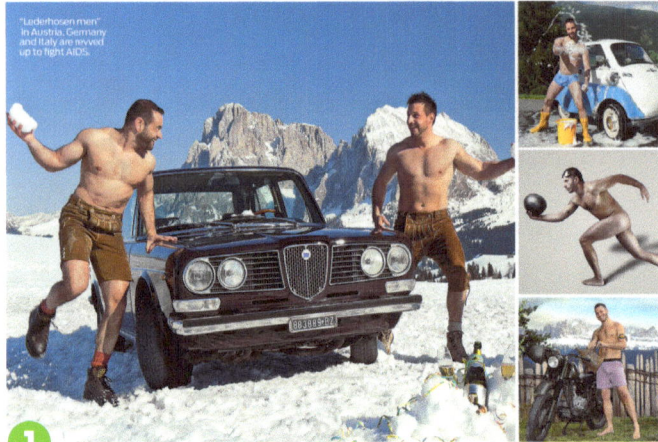

"Lederhosen men" in Austria, Germany and Italy are revved up to fight AIDS.

January/February

COVER: Linda and Nathaniel Scruggs and other couples living with HIV share their love stories. **INSIDE:** Debunking the misinformation about the rising rates of HIV among young African-American men who have sex with men; documentaries about the everyday heroes of the AIDS epidemic. **PLUS:** A charity calendar from the "Men in the Alps" (1).

March

COVER: Monica Thompson is grateful for the social services that have helped her stay in care. **INSIDE:** The executive director of AVAC outlines five priorities for action in biomedical HIV prevention; activists get naked to protest budget cuts. **PLUS:** A tribute to activist Spencer Cox (2).

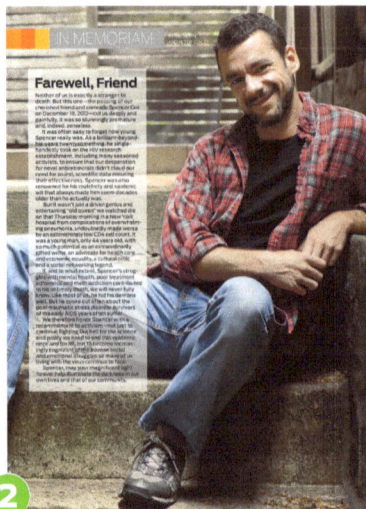

Farewell, Friend

April/May

COVER: *The Voice*'s Jamar Rogers shares his story about overcoming addiction (3). **INSIDE:** Navigating treatment as prevention in the real world; Alabama prisons end segregation for people living with HIV. **PLUS:** Reebok honors Keith Haring (4).

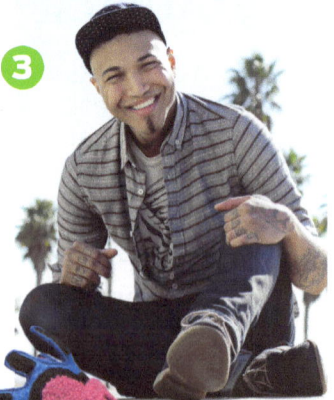

June

COVER: Mark S. King pens a powerful essay on why HIV stigma among gay men persists. **INSIDE:** Visual AIDS commemorates 25 years of art, AIDS and action (5); celebs sign up for an HBO movie version of *The Normal Heart*. **PLUS:** Is "the Mississippi Baby" the first child to be functionally cured of HIV?

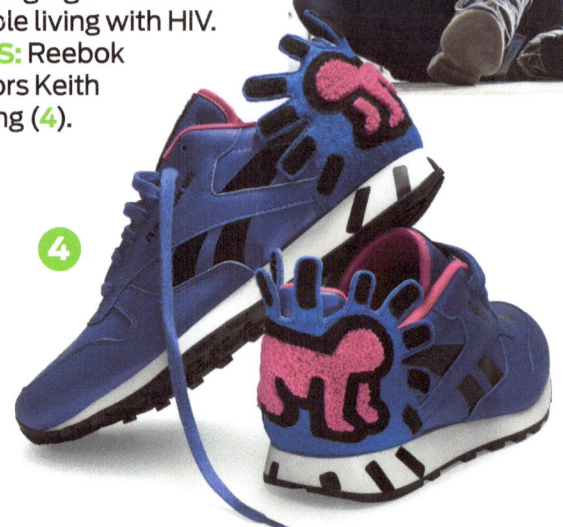

ART.AIDS.ACTION.

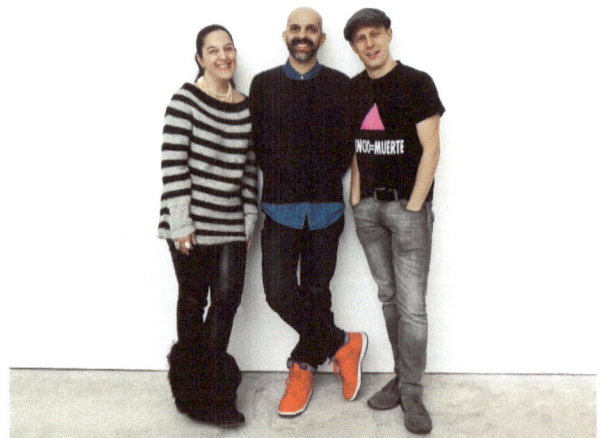

July/August

COVER: Our first-ever "negative" issue acknowledges the contributions of HIV-negative people, including Gwenn Barringer (on the cover with her HIV-positive husband, Shawn Decker). **INSIDE:** NMAC's Paul Kawata looks back at the early advocates in the fight; can barebacking be safer sex (6)? **PLUS:** New York City's Greenwich Village is getting an AIDS memorial.

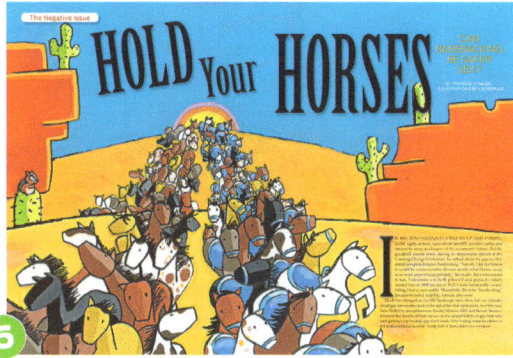

September

COVER: Three long-term survivors who have lived with HIV for more than 25 years share their survival savvy (7). **INSIDE:** People are facing delayed deliveries, spoiled shipments and privacy concerns with mail-order HIV meds (8). **PLUS:** Jewelry designer Rae Lewis-Thornton writes about how she deals with HIV one bead at a time.

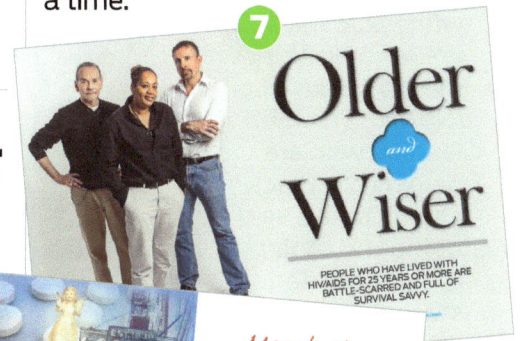

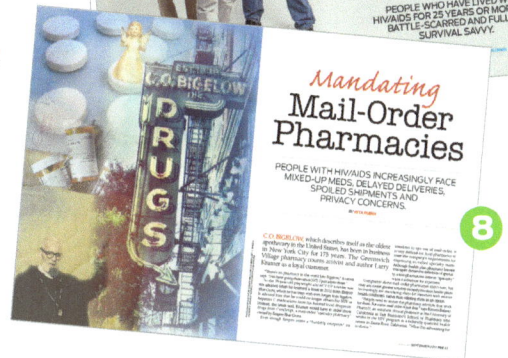

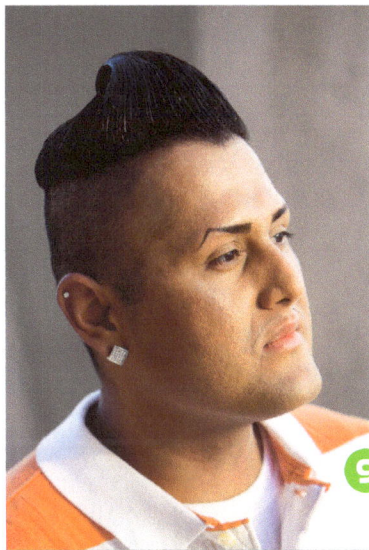

Older *and* Wiser

PEOPLE WHO HAVE LIVED WITH HIV/AIDS FOR 25 YEARS OR MORE ARE BATTLE-SCARRED AND FULL OF SURVIVAL SAVVY.

October/November

COVER: Daniel Leon's story is a reminder of the toll that Latino culture can take on the health of its people and raises the question: Are Latinos the next wave of the epidemic? (9). **INSIDE:** Meet Mr. Friendly, the new face of HIV awareness; can circumcision lower HIV rates in the United States? **PLUS:** Lower bone density linked to a number of antiretroviral regimens.

Mandating Mail-Order Pharmacies

PEOPLE WITH HIV/AIDS INCREASINGLY FACE MIXED-UP MEDS, DELAYED SHIPMENTS AND PRIVACY CONCERNS.

December

COVER: Shining a spotlight on 100 unsung heroes who are making a difference in the fight against HIV/AIDS. **INSIDE:** A roundtable of advocates living with HIV explore the role networks can play in fighting the virus (10). **PLUS:** Terrence McNally and Tyne Daly return to Broadway with the new AIDS-themed play *Mothers and Sons*.

Positive Networks

PEOPLE LIVING WITH HIV DISCUSS SELF-EMPOWERMENT.

ADVOCATES FROM A VARIETY OF NETWORKS of people living with HIV held a roundtable discussion earlier this year. The topic of the day was the networks themselves and the value they can have in our communities.

The roundtable, held in New York City at POZ headquarters, was based on the belief that people living with HIV should be full, active participants in the response against the epidemic and in decisions that affect them, be it within the positive community itself, on boards for local AIDS service organizations, or in governmental policy-making efforts.

This fundamental human rights concept is rooted in The Denver Principles, a self-empowerment manifesto written in 1983 by people living with HIV/AIDS. The idea was advanced at the 1994 Paris AIDS Summit with the GIPA (Greater

Involvement of People Living With HIV/AIDS) Principle.

Participants at the roundtable discussed the importance of networks in the lives of people living with HIV, the barriers to joining and expanding these networks, and the power such organizations can wield in addressing the epidemic.

In alphabetical order, the participants included: Deloris Dockrey, director of community organizing at the Hyacinth AIDS Foundation; Tami Haught, president of Positive Iowans Taking Charge; Jahlove Serrano, spokesmodel at Love Heals Speakers Bureau; Andrew R. Spieldenner, PhD, assistant professor at Hofstra University; Robert Suttle, assistant director at the Sero Project; and Reed Vreeland, communications coordinator at the Sero Project. The moderator was Laurel Sprague, research director at the Sero Project.

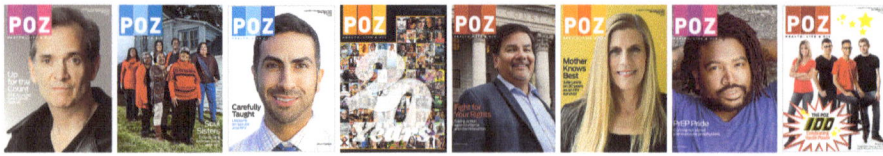

2014

January/February

COVER: POZ founder Sean Strub bears witness to the AIDS epidemic in his new memoir, *Body Counts*. **INSIDE:** The faith leaders who are helping the Black church take a seat at the HIV table; Republican-led states say no to Medicaid expansion, which affects people with HIV. **PLUS:** POZ pays tribute to Dennis Daniel, our dear friend and coworker (1).

March

COVER: The women of Common Threads reveal how an HIV intervention grew into a surprising microenterprise (2). **INSIDE:** Kathie Hiers of AIDS Alabama weighs in on the HIV epidemic in the South; the Stigma Index launches in the United States. **PLUS:** Living with HIV doesn't keep Jessica Whitbread from her art—or advocacy.

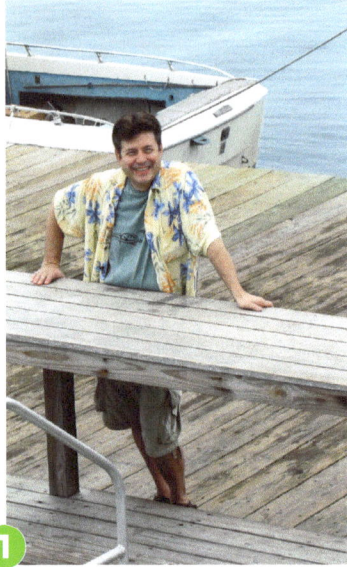

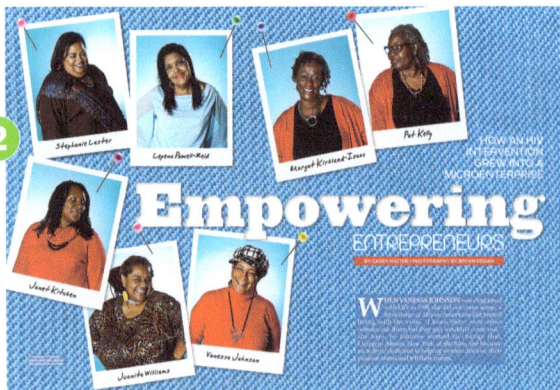

April/May

COVER: Jason Villalobos teaches HIV education in Santa Barbara, California. **INSIDE:** Playing the HIV numbers games is less—and more—risky than you think (3); condomless sex rises among gay men. **PLUS:** The CDC agrees to no longer use the term "unprotected sex" when it specifically means "sex without condoms."

June

COVER: POZ commemorates 20 years of empowering the HIV community. **INSIDE:** Twenty survivors from the covers of POZ share their stories and words of wisdom; catching up with Ty Ross, our first cover subject (4). **PLUS:** #TruvadaWhore T-shirts help to educate the public about PrEP.

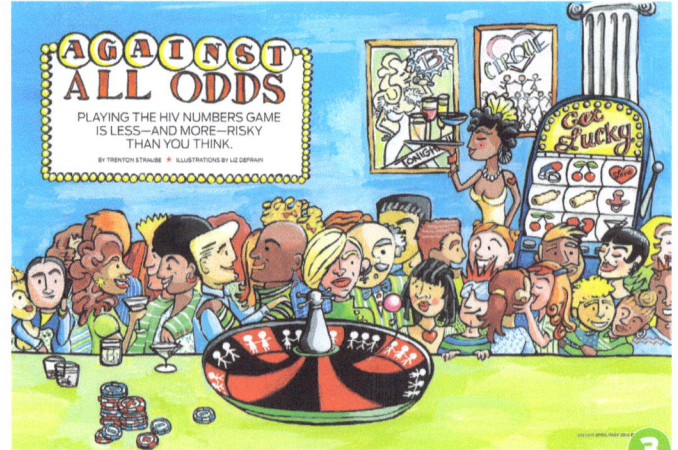

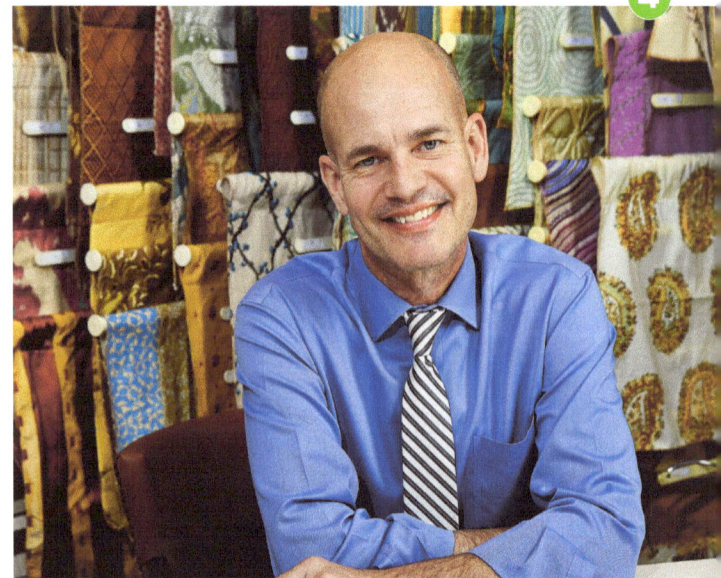

July/August

COVER: A jury awards Antonio Muñoz $500,000 for workplace discrimination. Learn how you can fight for your rights. **INSIDE:** Promising research suggests long-acting antiretrovirals may become a reality; how each of us can help fight HIV-related stigma (**5**). **PLUS:** Treatment Action Group's Tim Horn explains why new guidelines include cost considerations.

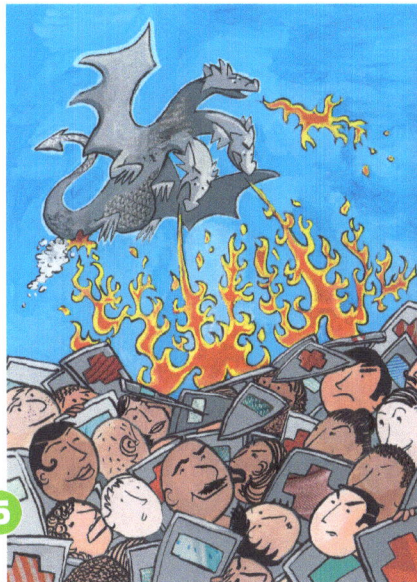

September

COVER: Julie Lewis and the 30/30 Project seek to build affordable health centers for those most in need (**6**). **INSIDE:** A new musical about disco legend Sylvester; "Start Talking. Stop HIV" is the CDC's latest HIV prevention campaign. **PLUS:** Activist Tez Anderson helps create the first HIV/AIDS Long-Term Survivors Awareness Day.

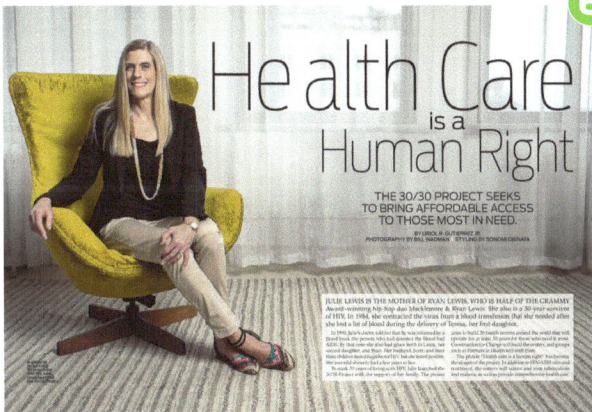

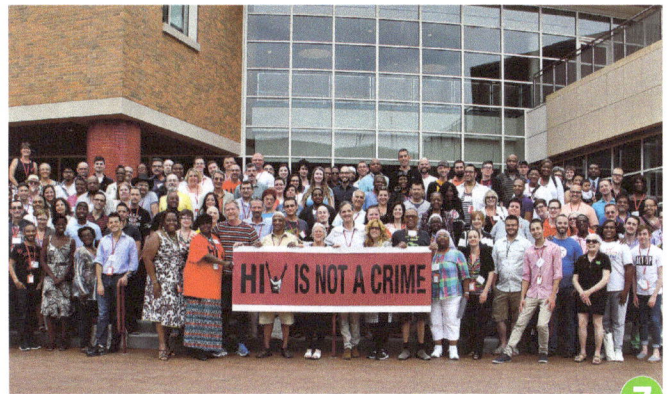

October/November

COVER: Quentin Ergane opens up about using PrEP to prevent HIV transmission. **INSIDE:** The nation's first HIV Is Not a Crime conference is held in Grinnell, Iowa (**7**); pharma giants team up for a new two-drug, single-tablet regimen to treat HIV. **PLUS:** The virus returns in "the Mississippi Baby," who had been thought to be functionally cured of HIV.

December

COVER: The POZ 100 celebrates youth power by highlighting 100 individuals under 30 who are fighting against HIV/AIDS. **INSIDE:** Texas fundraisers help people with AIDS get home for the holidays. **PLUS:** Olympic diver Greg Louganis reflects on making a documentary about his life (**8**).

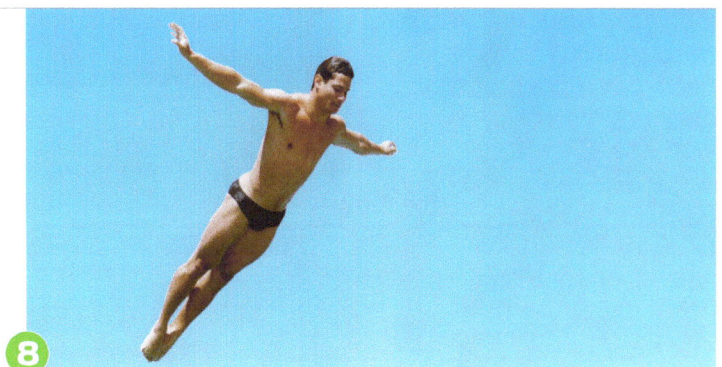

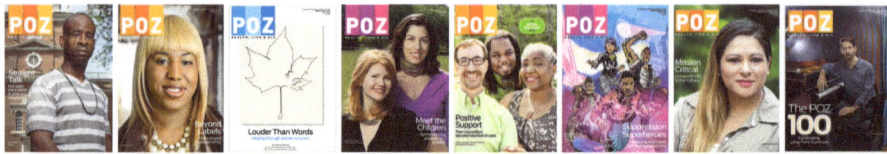

2015

April/May

COVER: A look at the work of artist Eric Rhein—including *Life Altering Spencer*, for AIDS activist Spencer Cox (1968–2012) (3). **INSIDE:** Poet Mary Bowman uses storytelling to educate others about HIV (4); an exclusive look at the exhibit *Art AIDS America*. **PLUS:** Photographer and activist Duane Cramer hopes to reduce stigma through his art.

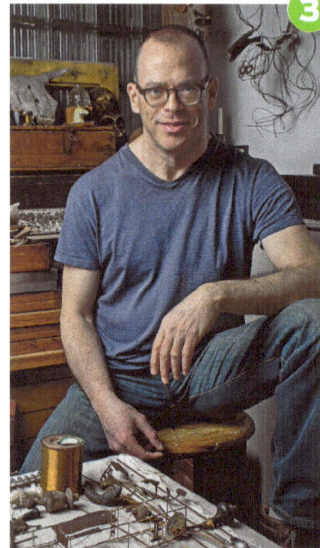
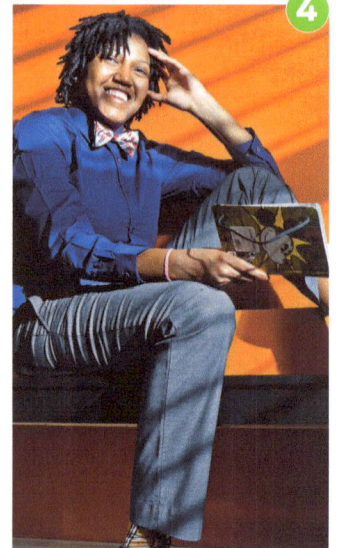

January/February

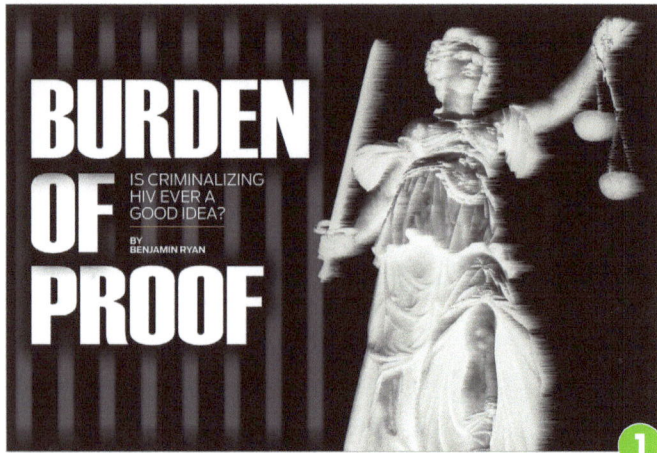

COVER: Benjamin Green, an advocate for peer education programs in and out of prison, helps straight men who have HIV. **INSIDE:** Venton Jones hopes to bring HIV issues to the National Black Justice Coalition; is criminalizing HIV ever a good idea (1)? **PLUS:** AIDS and Ebola: History repeats itself.

June

COVER: Whitney Joiner and Alysia Abbott each lost a parent to AIDS and started the Recollectors, a group to support others like themselves. **INSIDE:** Mark S. King's essay on his relevance as a long-term HIV survivor (5). **PLUS:** GMHC CEO Kelsey Louie talks about his first year on the job.

March

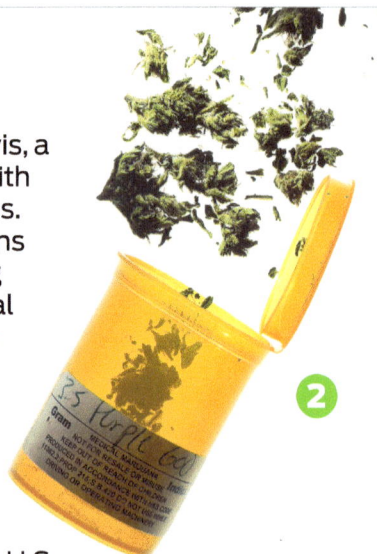

COVER: Octavia Lewis, a trans activist living with HIV, transcends labels. **INSIDE:** As ELISA turns 30, better HIV testing becomes more crucial as prevention efforts increase; the future of medical marijuana for HIV looks hazy (2); Gina Brown speaks up for HIV-positive Southern Black women. **PLUS:** U.S. treatment cascade stats.

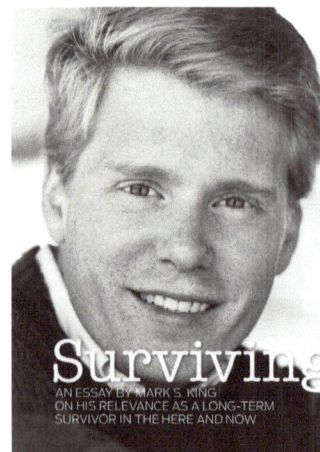
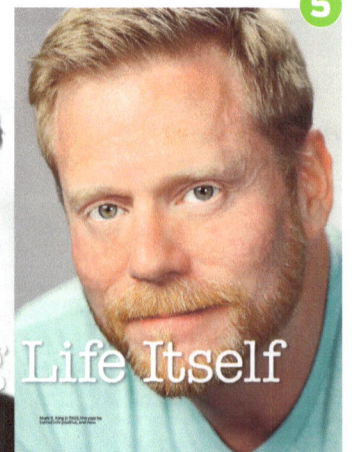

Surviving Life Itself
AN ESSAY BY MARK S. KING ON HIS RELEVANCE AS A LONG-TERM SURVIVOR IN THE HERE AND NOW

September

COVER: London Gray, Benjamin Ball, Adonis Porch and Ervin Rogers provide real-life inspiration for their comic-book counterparts in Housing Works' *The Undetectables* (**7**). **INSIDE:** New treatment options for people living with HIV and hepatitis C. **PLUS:** An archive of portraits and oral histories document the graying of AIDS.

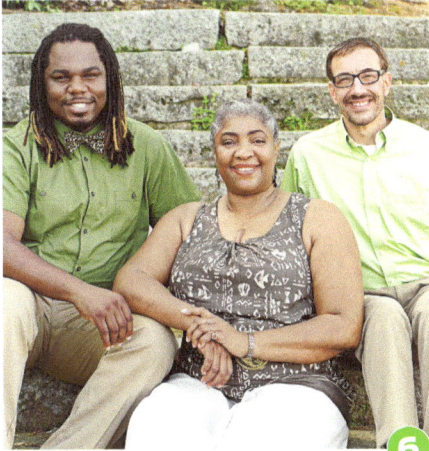

July/August

COVER: HIV-positive peer counselors Andrew Ballard, Tommy Williams and Debra Richards elevate retention in care in the South (**6**). **INSIDE:** Questioning the use of taxpayer funding for faith-based groups to fight AIDS; Marco Castro-Bojorquez is starting a national network for Latinos. **PLUS:** Robin Webb empowers peers in Mississippi.

October/November

COVER: Heather Arculeo—a former Marine who was discharged after testing HIV positive—and others discuss HIV and military service. **INSIDE:** Cutting through the hype and hyperbole to find the truth about HIV cure research (**8**); Moisés Agosto fights for minority groups. **PLUS:** Mondo Guerra on life after disclosing his status on *Project Runway*.

December

COVER: The sixth annual POZ 100 list celebrates long-term survivors who became HIV positive in 1995 or earlier. **INSIDE:** A Q&A with renowned jazz pianist and composer Fred Hersch; WHO focuses on the needs of transgender people. **PLUS:** Longtime activist Jim Eigo, reminds us long-term survivors can be HIV positive or negative (**9**).

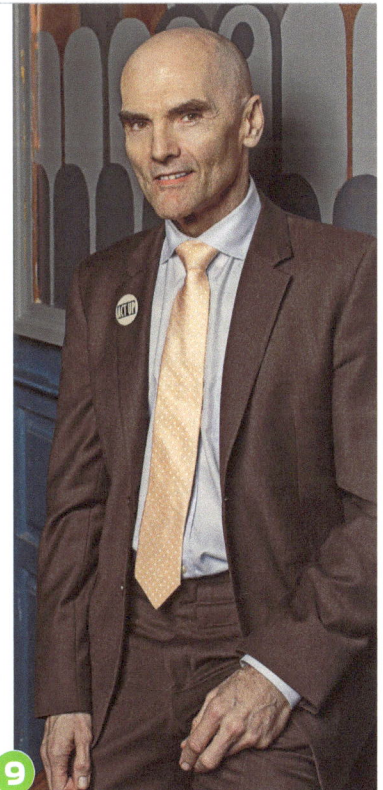

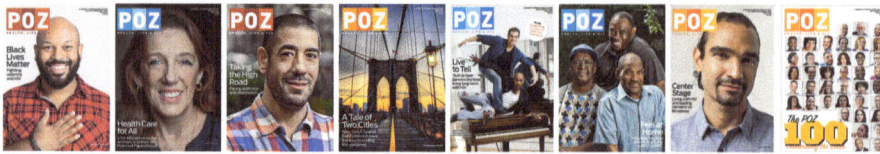

2016

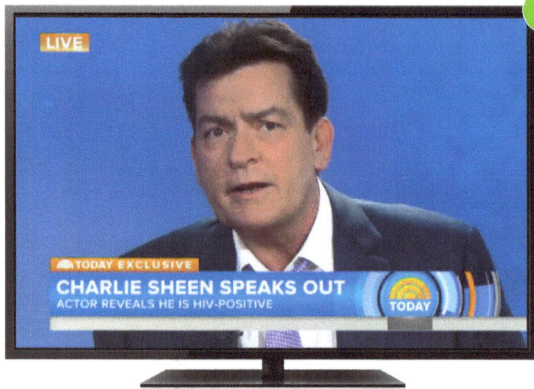

January/February

COVER: Ashton P. Woods and other Black activists are finding common cause in fighting violence and HIV. **INSIDE:** After his public disclosure, Charlie Sheen puts HIV in the news again (1); navigating sex and disclosure while living with HIV. **PLUS:** Activists protest after Martin Shkreli of Turing Pharmaceuticals raises the price of an AIDS-related drug by 5,000%.

March

COVER: Nancy Duncan is a peer educator for Planned Parenthood and sees firsthand the vital HIV services the group provides for women and men (2). **INSIDE:** Strut, an HIV and wellness center, opens in San Francisco; the first single-tablet combo with the new tenofovir gets the green light from the FDA. **PLUS:** Share your thoughts on clinical trials in the POZ survey.

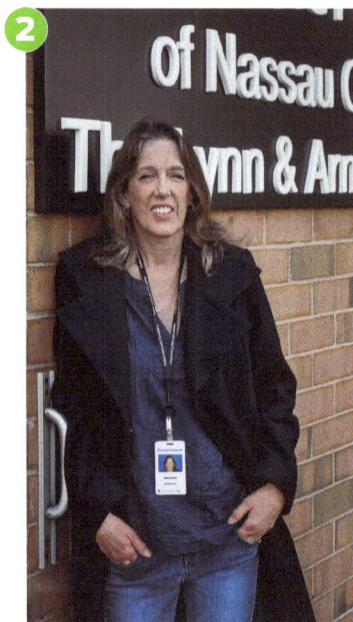

April/May

COVER: Anthony Romano shares his story and reminds us why crystal meth still attracts gay men. **INSIDE:** Depression is often a silent partner to HIV; HBO's *Mapplethorpe: Look at the Pictures* reveals the man behind the camera and the controversy (3). **PLUS:** Elizabeth Taylor's grand-kids participate in AIDSWatch to promote comprehensive sex education.

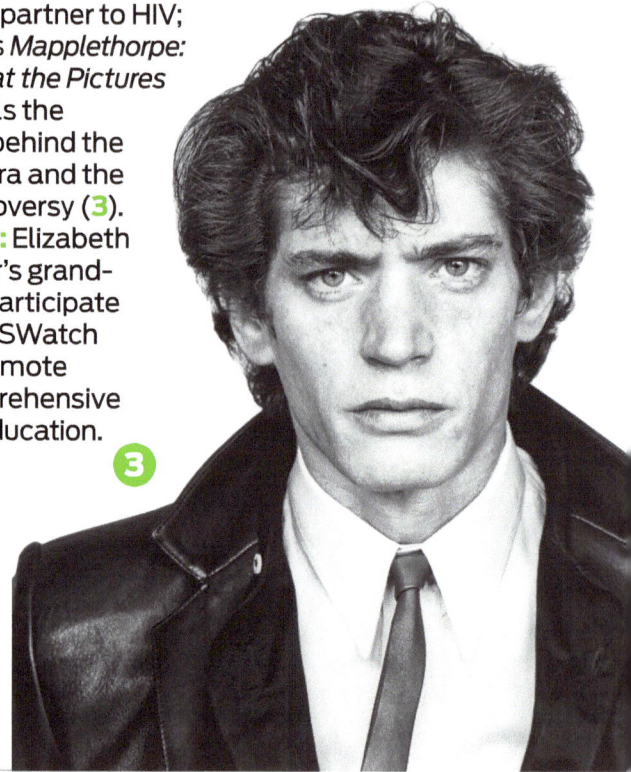

June

COVER: San Francisco and New York City pave the way to ending the HIV epidemic (4). **INSIDE:** America addresses its opioid addiction; an HIV treatment taken only every two months moves closer to reality. **PLUS:** Olympic gold medalist Greg Louganis finally gets his box of Wheaties.

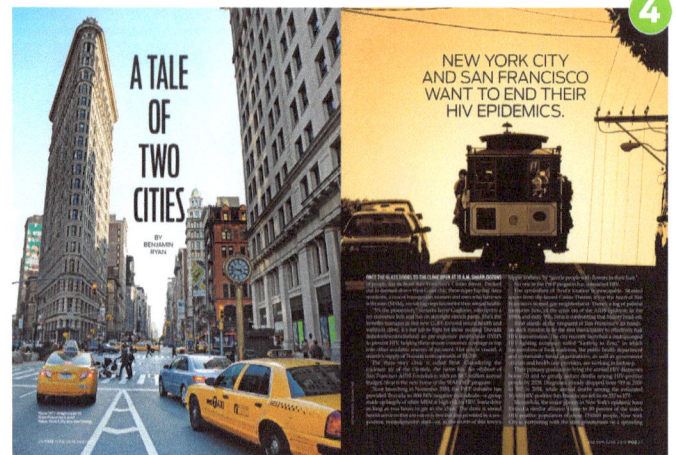

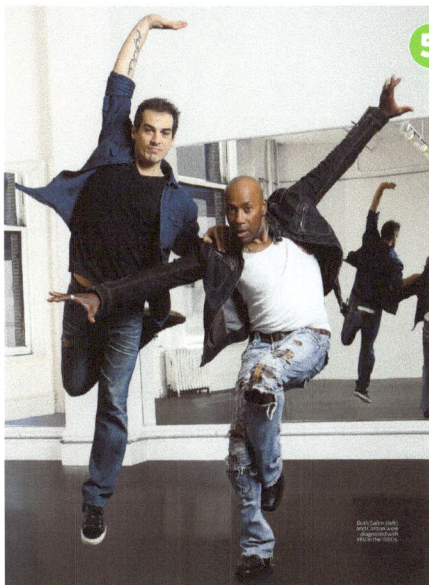

July/August

COVER: Salim "Slam" Gauwloos and Carlton Wilborn shine the spotlight on HIV in a new film about Madonna's Blond Ambition tour dancers (**5**). **INSIDE:** *Desert Migration* profiles long-term survivors in Palm Springs, California; Doug Meyer creates sculptures of creative icons lost to AIDS. **PLUS:** An excerpt from Tim Murphy's novel *Christodora*, about the early (and future) years of the epidemic in New York.

September

COVER: Alfred Baker, Clifton Alford and John Lawton on the importance of finding housing solutions for older Americans living with HIV (**6**). **INSIDE:** The Reunion Project gives long-term survivors the chance to tell their stories about loss and life; social media stars use their platforms for HIV prevention. **PLUS:** Can supervised injection facilities help reduce HIV and hepatitis C rates in the United States?

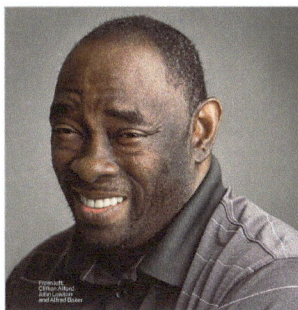
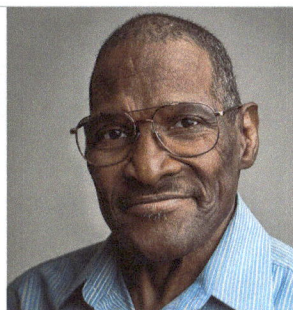
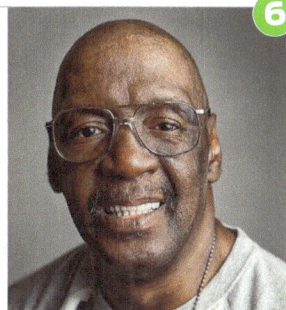

FINDING SOLUTIONS TO HOUSING OLDER AMERICANS LIVING WITH HIV/AIDS

Feel at Home

October/ November

COVER: Javier Muñoz on living with HIV and starring as Hamilton on Broadway (**7**). **INSIDE:** How national, state and local elections will affect HIV prevention; undetectable equals untransmittable messaging grows stronger after the latest results from the PARTNER study. **PLUS:** A front-row seat at GMHC's Latex Ball.

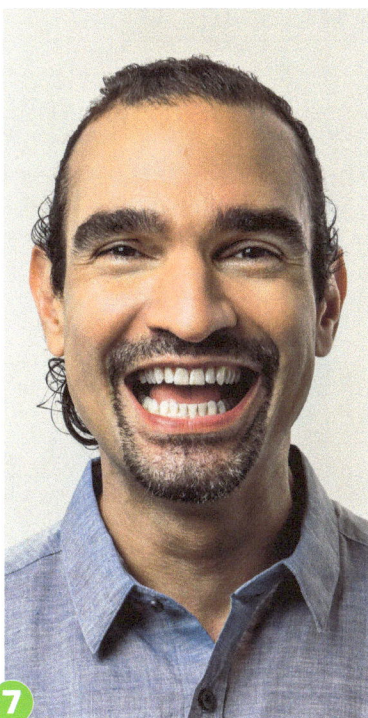

December

COVER: Our 7th annual POZ 100 showcases people living and working in the South who are making a difference in the fight against HIV/AIDS. **INSIDE:** The director of *Wilhemina's War* reflects on the struggles of people living with HIV in the South; a viral photo campaign hopes to end stigma one portrait at a time (**8**). **PLUS:** Women living with HIV are "organizing for power" at Speak Up! 2016.

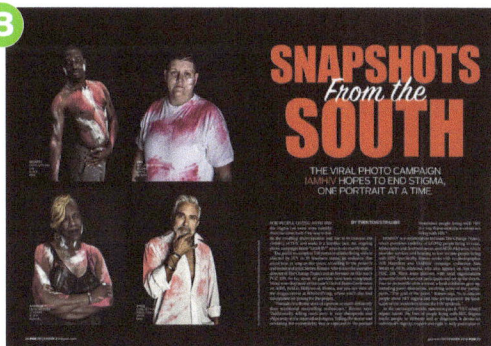

SNAPSHOTS *From the* SOUTH

THE VIRAL PHOTO CAMPAIGN IAMHIV HOPES TO END STIGMA, ONE PORTRAIT AT A TIME

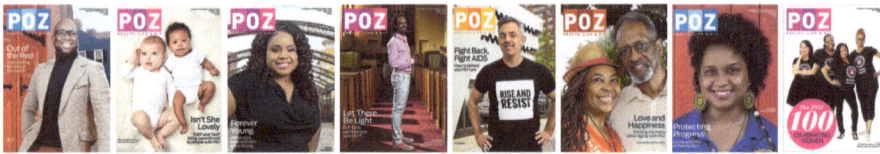

THE YEAR IN POZ

2017

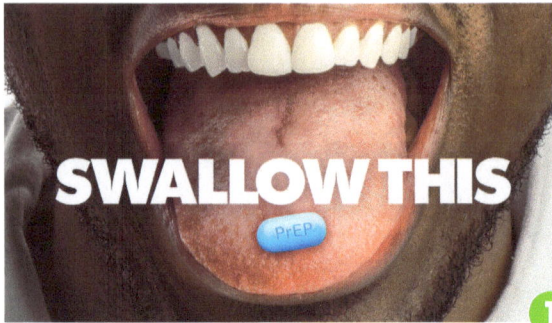

January/February

COVER: Marvell L. Terry II discusses the challenges facing Black gay and bisexual men at the center of the HIV/AIDS epidemic in the South. **INSIDE:** Is PrEP (pre-exposure prophylaxis) failing to reach those at highest risk for the virus? (**1**); the U.S. surgeon general endorses harm reduction strategies to treat addiction. **PLUS:** Queen front man Freddie Mercury shares the spotlight with the AIDS epidemic in a new biography, *Somebody to Love.*

March

COVER: HIV-negative babies like Mila Vreeland and Memory Amya Hunte dispel misconceptions about conception and HIV.
INSIDE: Buddy

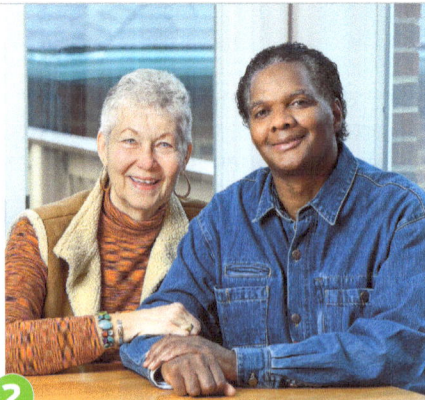

programs offer one-on-one support as they help people living with HIV tackle stigma and isolation (**2**); the advocacy group WORLD (Women Organized to Respond to Life-threatening Disease) commemorates its 25th anniversary. **PLUS:** The web comedy series *Mess* follows a group of best friends as they navigate love, lust and the virus in today's gay scene.

April/May

COVER: Our special gatefold cover features youth advocates Jake Glaser, Hydeia Broadbent, and siblings Alee, Mitchell and Yonas Meredith—all born with HIV and previously featured on a POZ cover (**3**). **INSIDE:** The @the_aids_memorial Instagram account is a touching visual tribute to lives lost to AIDS; Carl Siciliano founded the Ali Forney Center to help homeless LGBT youth. **PLUS:** The link between youth homelessness and HIV in the United States.

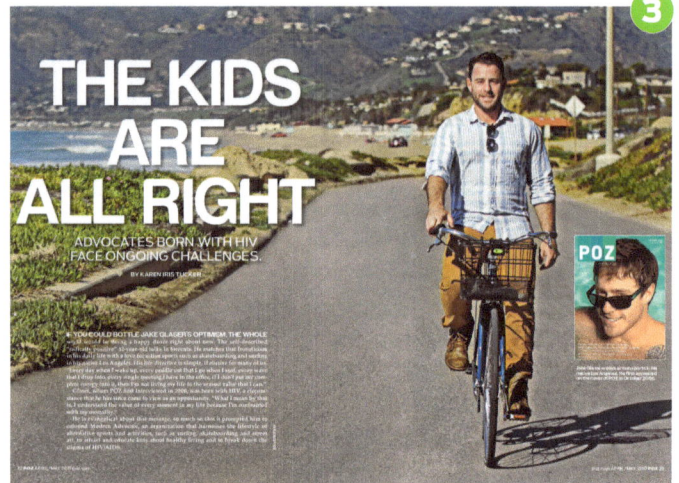

June

COVER: Minister Rob Newells is an African-American gay man living with HIV and working to build bridges between his communities. **INSIDE:** The aftermath of the Pulse nightclub mass shooting a year later; Jesse Milan of AIDS United shares his views on policy priorities for HIV advocacy. **PLUS:** How the legendary AIDS activist Larry Kramer made his way back to GMHC (**4**).

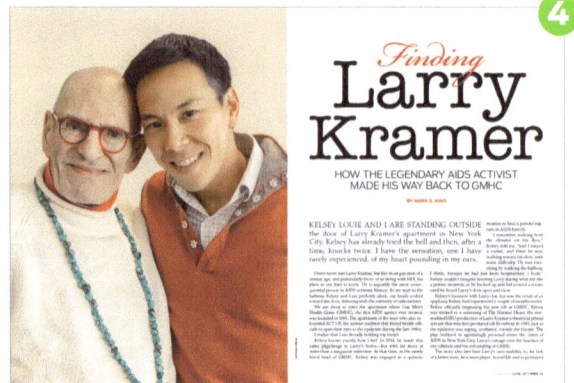

July/August

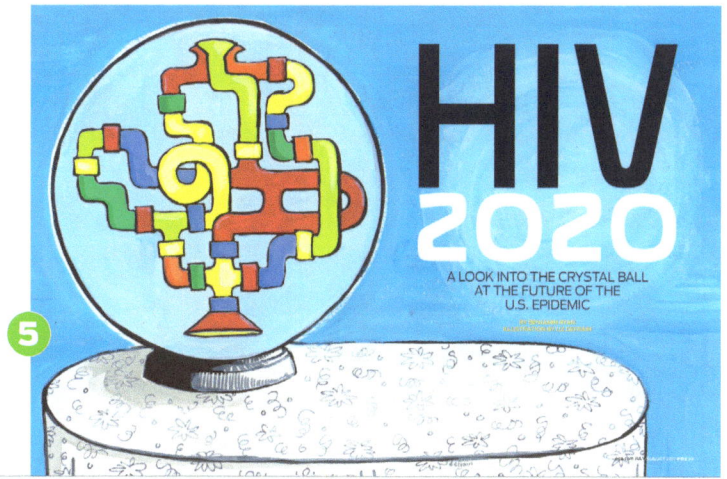

COVER: Tim Murphy and other activists living with HIV are fighting for their rights—and yours. **INSIDE:** Experts in the field weigh in on what the next decade of the HIV epidemic will look like (**5**); a U=U dance party in New York City. **PLUS:** 10 simple ways to fight the virus every day.

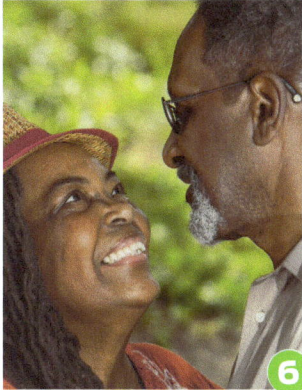

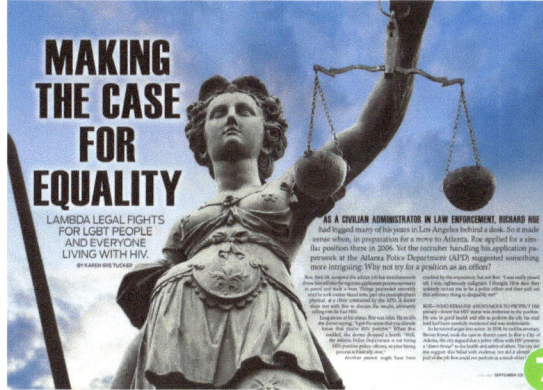

September

COVER: Anna Fowlkes (with partner Paul Johns) reminds us that aging with HIV doesn't have to mean living without love (**6**). **INSIDE:** Stephen Barker's portraits show early AIDS activists—minus the anger; Lambda Legal fights for LGBT people and everyone living with HIV (**7**). **PLUS:** The photography book *Dogs & Daddies* raises funds to help youth living with HIV.

October/November

COVER: Although the economic crisis in Puerto Rico threatens critical progress on HIV, L'Orangelis Thomas Negrón, Anselmo Fonseca (pictured below) and others are fighting back (**8**). **INSIDE:** HIV scientists and advocates are waging an effective war against the epidemic despite cutbacks and flat funding. **PLUS:** The exhibit *AIDS at Home: Art and Everyday Activism* explores hidden stories of the epidemic.

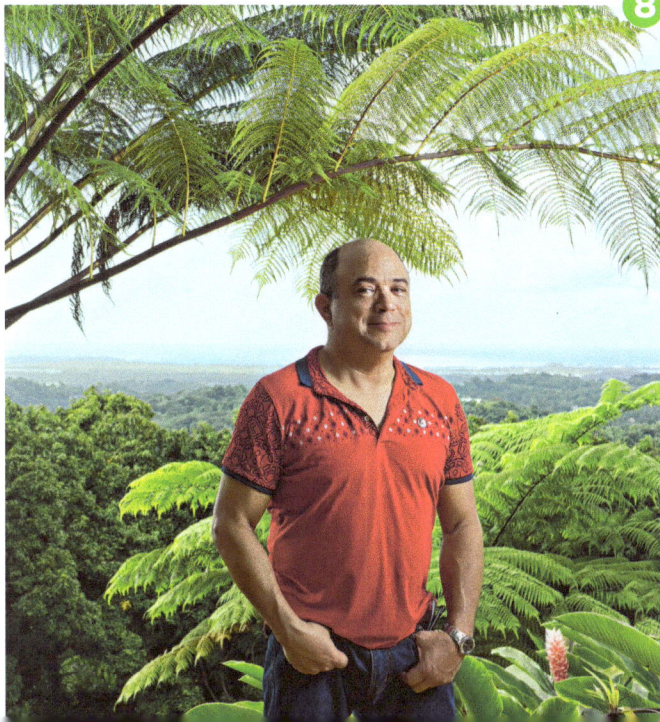

December

COVER: Our gatefold cover features advocates from the Positive Women's Network–USA. They're a handful of the women living with HIV highlighted in this year's POZ 100 (**9**). **INSIDE:** Immigration Equality advocates on behalf of both LGBT immigrants and those living with HIV; highlights from the United States Conference on AIDS in Washington, DC. **PLUS:** Visual AIDS commissions seven videos of Black narratives on the epidemic for this year's Day With(Out) Art.

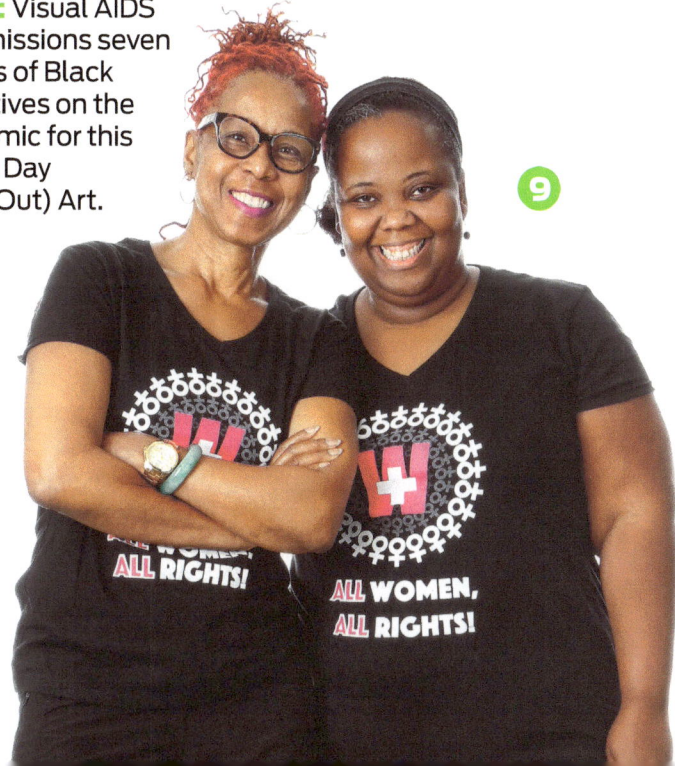

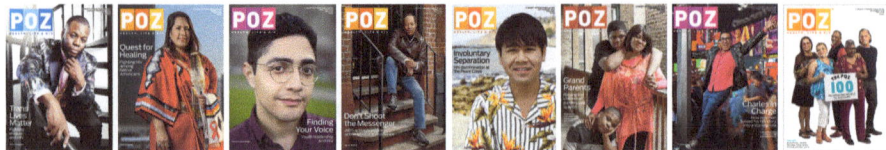

THE YEAR IN POZ
2018

January/February

COVER: Achim Howard and other trans advocates stormed the stage at USCA to express their frustration with the omission of trans people (1). **INSIDE:** French director Robin Campillo goes behind the scenes of his ACT UP Paris film, *BPM (Beats Per Minute)*. **PLUS:** An excerpt of Avram Finkelstein's new book recounts how "Silence= Death" became a rallying cry for ACT UP.

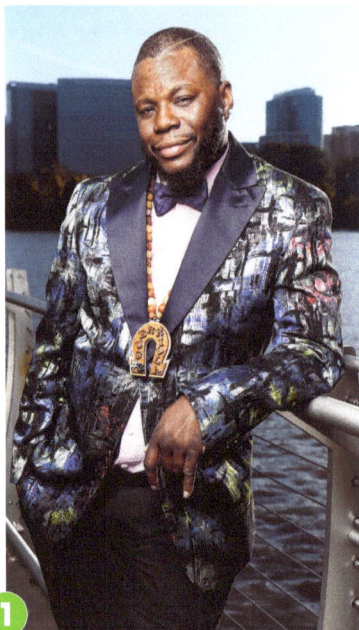

March

COVER: Native American Shana Cozad has reached a truce with her virus, thanks to the healing power of her tribe's spiritual advisers (2). **INSIDE:** How groups of women living with HIV are expanding their reach; the FDA approves the first HIV treatment containing only two antiretrovirals. **PLUS:** 10 simple ways to fight HIV every day.

April/May

COVER: Advocate Giuliani Alvarenga seeks support for youth leaders to better address HIV among Latinos. **INSIDE:** Mark S. King explores why there are still so many AIDS-related deaths (3); why PrEP has an uncertain future among youth under 25. **PLUS:** Tony Kushner's *Angels in America* returns to Broadway after 25 years.

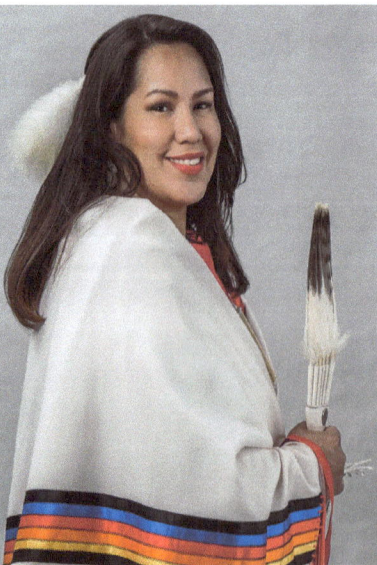

June

COVER: Jay W. Walker, a long-term HIV survivor, links past AIDS activism to current efforts to prevent gun violence (4). **INSIDE:** A look at AIDSWatch 2018; artist Nelson Santos showcases the powerful bond between people and their pets. **PLUS:** Meet President Trump's controversial new director of the CDC.

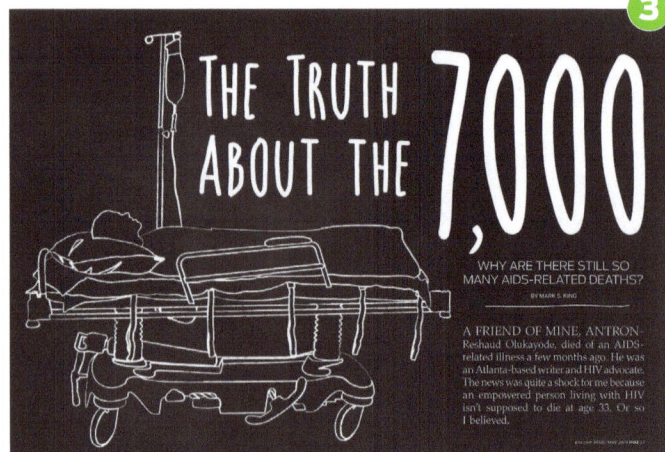

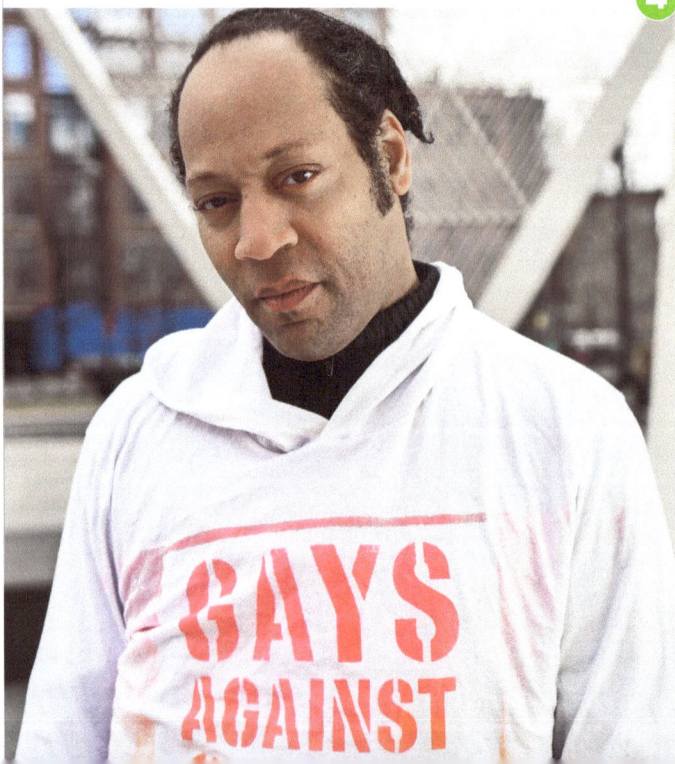

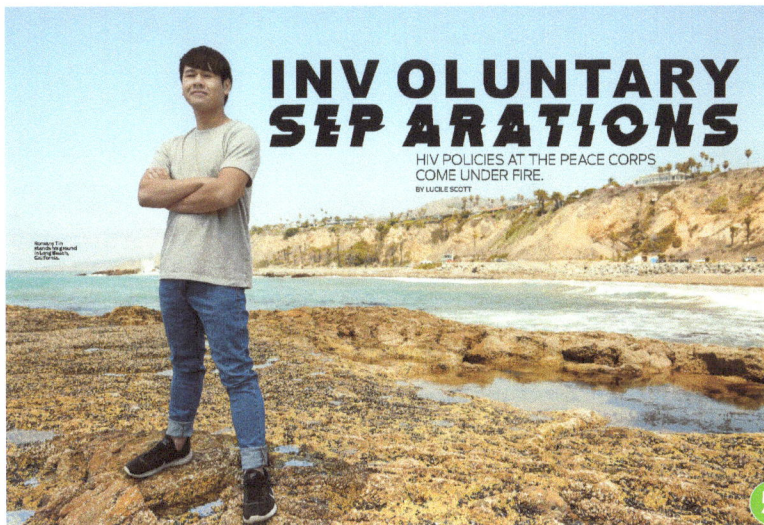

July/August

COVER: After testing HIV positive, Romany Tin was discharged from his post as a Peace Corps volunteer (5). **INSIDE:** Why curing hep C is a priority for people also living with HIV; the FDA approves three new, cheaper antiretroviral combination tablets. **PLUS:** Nelson Vergel advocates for the development of new salvage therapies.

September

COVER: Nora Young raises her two HIV-negative grandchildren after the 2013 death of her daughter, who was living with the virus. **INSIDE:** POZ interviews the new executive director of Visual AIDS, Esther McGowan; Life Ball, the annual lavish fundraiser in Vienna, commemorates its 25th anniversary (6). **PLUS:** The latest CDC campaign launches with new faces and a timeless message.

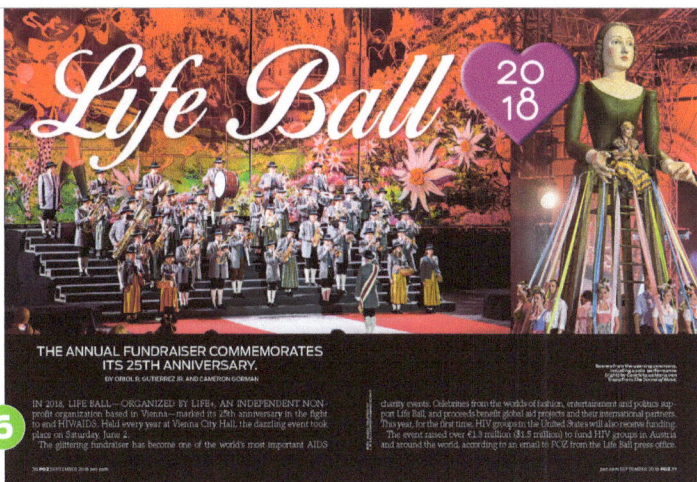

October/November

COVER: Actor Charles Sanchez shares with POZ how his HIV journey inspired his hit web series, *Merce.* **INSIDE:** Understanding the connections between sex work and HIV; POZ explores the impact of Hurricane Maria on people with HIV in Puerto Rico. **PLUS:** Contestants strike a pose at GMHC's annual Latex Ball in New York City (7).

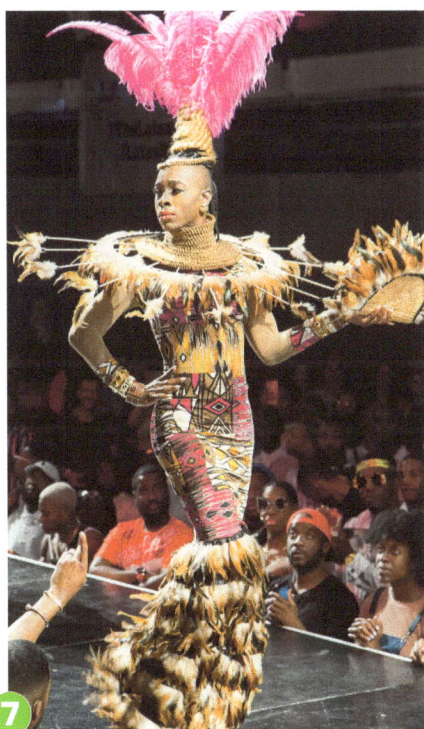

December

COVER: The 2018 POZ 100 list celebrates advocates living with HIV who are 50 and over (8). **INSIDE:** A Q&A with Moisés Agosto-Rosario, treatment director of NMAC (National Minority AIDS Council); an oral history of AIDS and art; a social media recap of USCA 2018; everyday milestones in the epidemic. **PLUS:** Longtime advocate Krishna Stone celebrates 25 years at Gay Men's Health Crisis.

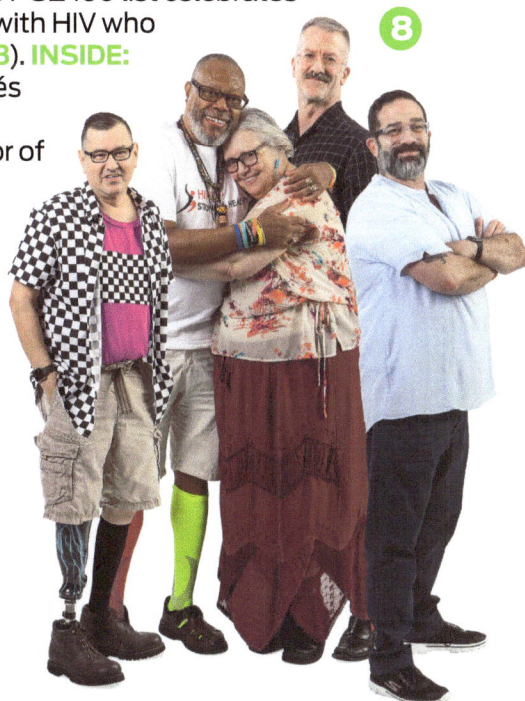

2019

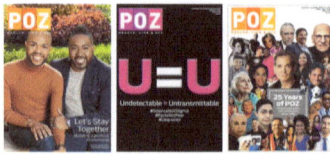

January/February

COVER: Serodiscordant couple (and Atlanta-based advocates) David Massey (left) and Johnny Lester are committed to each other—and to overcoming challenges to their union (**1**). **INSIDE:** Portraits of AIDS activists in a new book by photographer and ACT UP member Bill Bytsura (**2**); the road ahead for HIV cure research. **PLUS:** #LivingwithHIVwhileBlack by blogger Aundaray Guess.

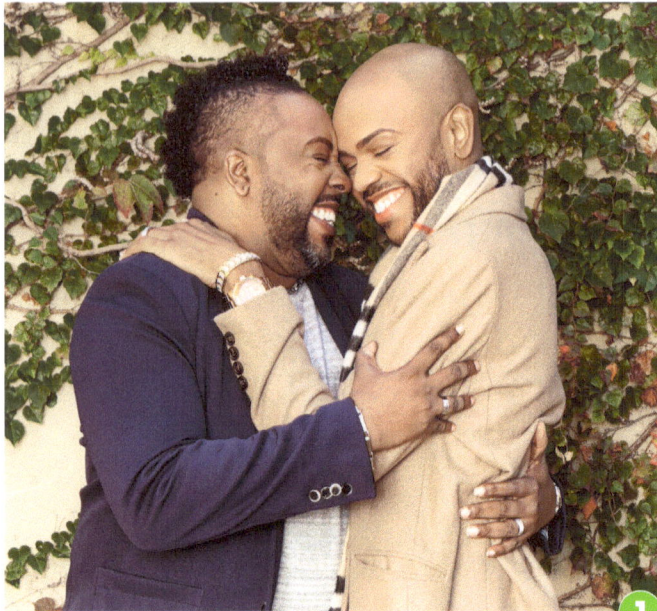

March

COVER: Understanding the undetectable equals untransmittable (U=U) movement, plus a pullout poster with tips for communicating the message (**3**). **INSIDE:** Why it's important to ensure health equity for all people living with HIV, regardless of viral load; the winners of the 2018 POZ Awards. **PLUS:** A Q&A with Raniyah Copeland, the new president and CEO of the Black AIDS Institute.

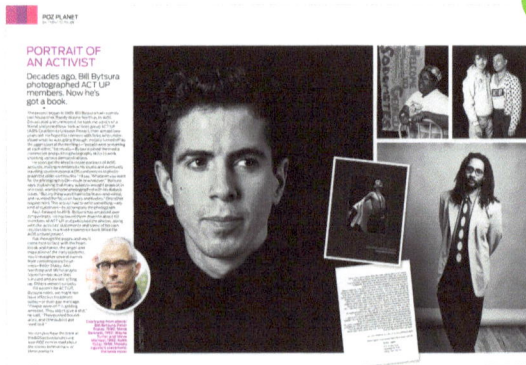

April/May

COVER: The 25th anniversary issue of POZ features a gatefold cover showing a collage of many folks who have graced the cover since 1994 (**4**). **INSIDE:** Catching up with 25 advocates featured on the POZ cover; a profile on POZ founder Sean Strub. **PLUS:** A very, very brief history of HIV.

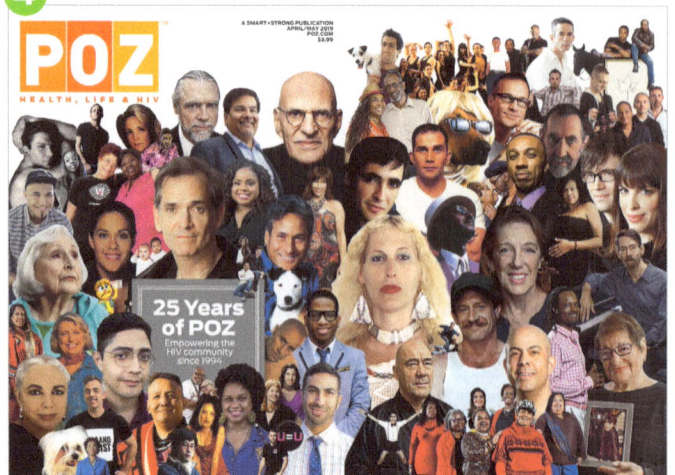

POZ EN ESPAÑOL

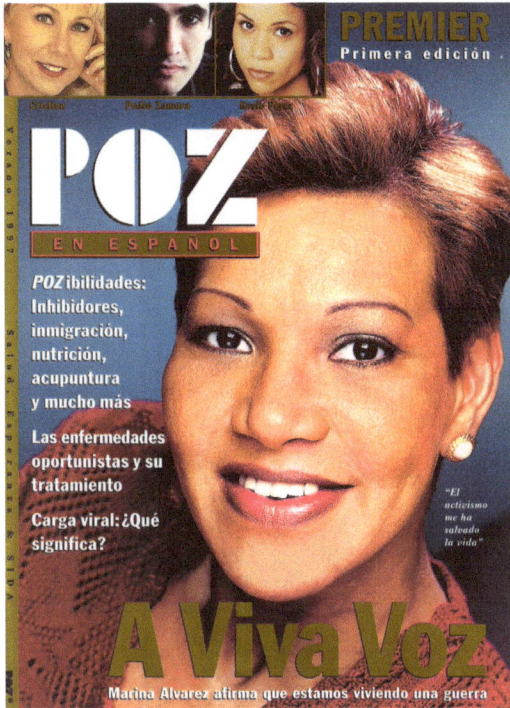
Verano 1997

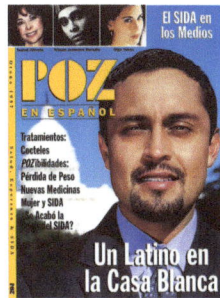
Otoño 1997

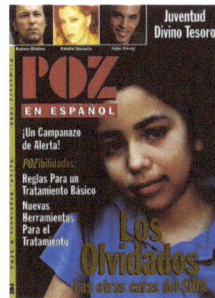
Primavera 1998

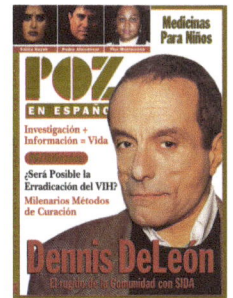
Verano 1998

The Spanish-language version of POZ, created with all original content, launched in 1997. Although it folded in 2003 because of a lack of advertising support, the magazine was well received.

La versión en español de la revista POZ, creada con todo el contenido original, se lanzó en 1997. La revista fue bien recibida, a pesar de que en 2003 dejó de publicarse por falta de apoyo publicitario.

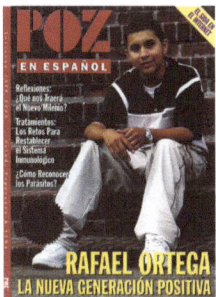
Invierno 1999/2000

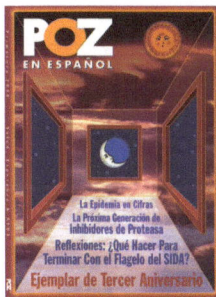
Primavera 2000

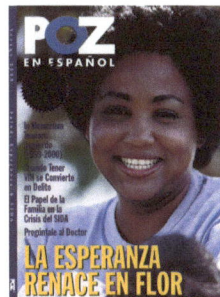
Verano 2000

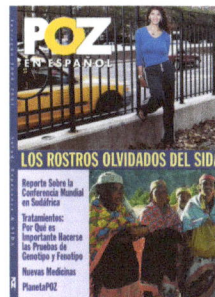
Invierno 2000/2001

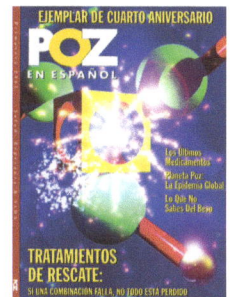
Primavera 2001

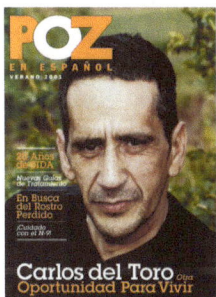
Verano 2001

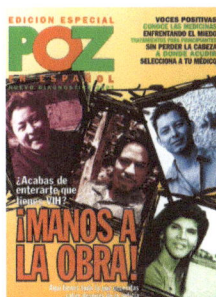
Edición Especial 2001

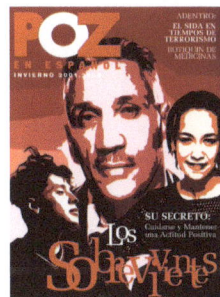
Invierno 2001/2002

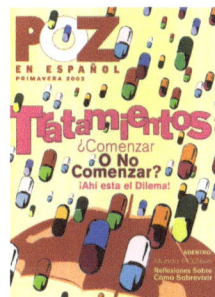
Primavera 2002

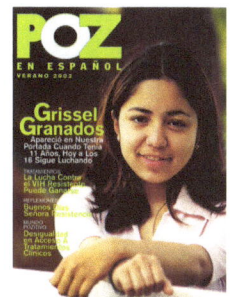
Invierno 2002

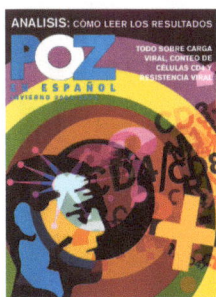
Invierno 2002/2003

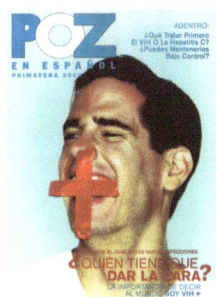
Primavera 2003

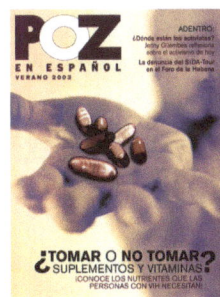
Verano 2003

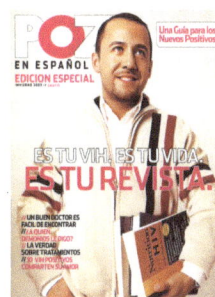
Edición Especial 2003

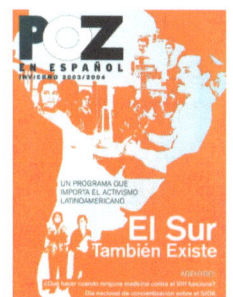
Invierno 2003/2004

POZ.COM

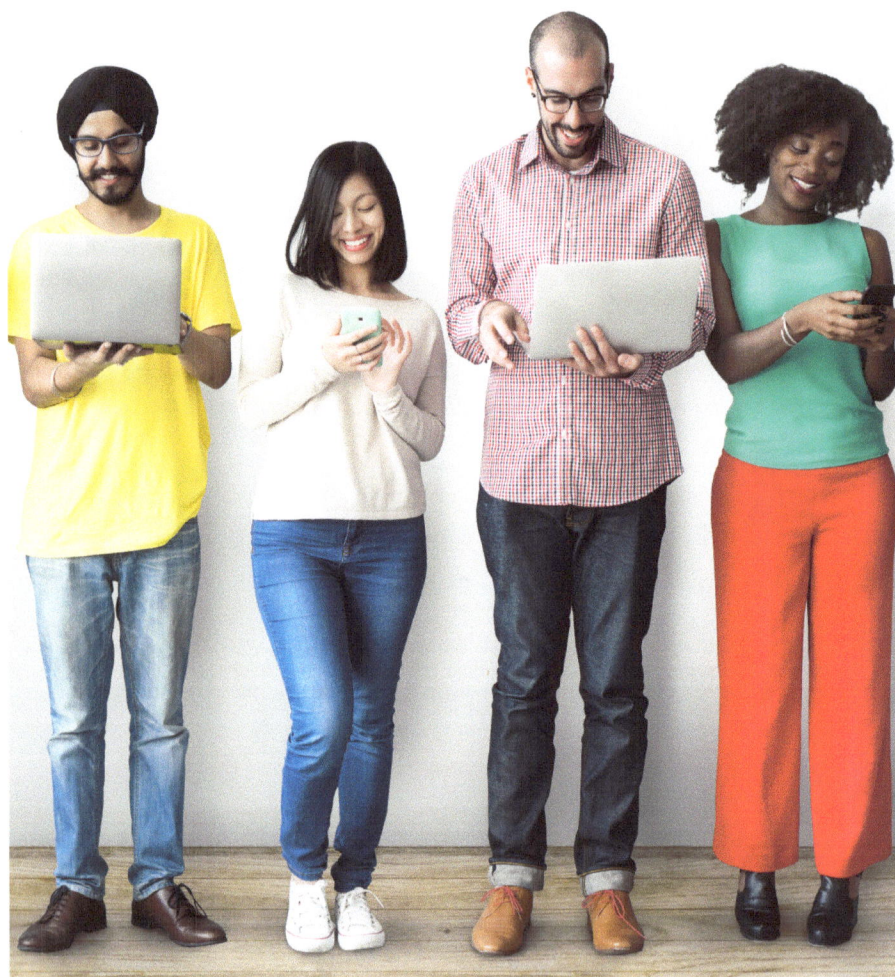

LAUNCHED IN 1996, POZ.COM PROVIDES AN ARCHIVE of every issue of POZ magazine. The site also posts daily national and international HIV/AIDS news, treatment updates and special reports on a wide variety of cultural, social, political and medical topics. POZ.com also offers members of the HIV community opportunities to come together to share their stories, experiences and expertise through a variety of web and social media platforms.

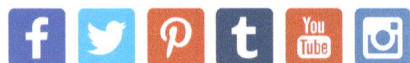

POZ News
Up-to-date information on an array of topics related to HIV

POZ Blogs
Insights from a diverse group of bloggers on a variety of issues

POZ Stories
The real-life stories of people living with and affected by HIV/AIDS

POZ Archive
Access to every print issue from the past 25 years

POZ Personals
The premier online dating service for people living with HIV

POZ Forums
A round-the-clock discussion area for people concerned about HIV/AIDS

Basics
Essential information about HIV testing, transmission, prevention, treatment and more

Conference Coverage
The latest HIV-related news and highlights from conferences around the world

Health Services Directory
A comprehensive and searchable guide to health care and services for people with HIV

Calendar
A listing of upcoming events relevant to the HIV community

Life After POZ

In 1994, frustrated by the media's coverage of the AIDS epidemic, activist Sean Strub started a magazine to amplify the voices of people living with HIV. He named it POZ.

"Almost no one knew what 'POZ' meant when we launched," Strub recalls. "It had the advantage of serving as a double entendre, meaning both 'HIV positive' as well as 'thinking positive and taking control of one's life,' which was central to the magazine's message."

Many people at the time doubted that POZ would last. But Strub, who tested HIV positive in 1985, had sold his insurance policies and invested everything he had into the start-up, which was produced in his New York City loft.

"When I was really sick, POZ gave me a purpose that was crystal clear," he says. "That purpose was important to my survival during a time when I might just as easily have died."

Strub served as publisher and executive editor of POZ until he sold the magazine in 2004, at which point he relocated to Milford, Pennsylvania, a small town he grew fond of in the late '90s.

Milford also piqued his interest in historic preservation. "Twenty years later, I've restored or improved 20 buildings and helped launch festivals, a community foundation and other endeavors," Strub says.

One of the buildings he renovated was the Hotel Fauchère. In 2001, Strub and a partner acquired the defunct landmark hotel. Five years later, it reopened for business. The hotel continues to operate today with Strub as owner.

He recently created the Hotel Fauchère Fund to help support local charitable efforts.

But Strub's most important role in Milford is serving as its mayor. In 2016, he was unanimously appointed mayor by the town's council before getting elected by its residents the following year.

Strub is no stranger to politics. He was the first openly HIV-positive person to run for U.S. Congress in 1990, and he details his candidacy in his 2014 autobiography, *Body Counts: A Memoir of Politics, Sex, AIDS, and Survival*.

His mayoral responsibilities notwithstanding, Strub still advocates for people living with HIV.

He is the executive director of the Sero Project, a network of people living with HIV working to fight stigma and HIV criminalization. The group produces the biennial HIV Is Not a Crime Training Academy as well as a health and wellness resource guide for prisoners with HIV and hepatitis.

"I have learned so much and become a better person through my work with other people with HIV, and that is no different today than it was 25 years ago," he says.

Strub's advice to people living with HIV is: Make connections, be of service and have hope.

As for POZ commemorating its silver anniversary, Strub is proud of "the community of people living with HIV, our closest friends and allies who have helped sustain the magazine and carry forth the values we espouse to a broader world." —ALICIA GREEN

Sean Strub is the founder of POZ and mayor of Milford, Pennsylvania.

BILL WADMAN

AFTERWORD

THERE ARE COUNTLESS PEOPLE TO THANK FOR THE CONTINUING WORK OF POZ, BUT HERE'S A LIST OF THE STAFF AND freelancers who have appeared on the past 25 years of mastheads, in alphabetical order:

John A. Adames, Manu Aggarwal, Doug Allen, Johnetta A. Alston, Robert Arthur Altman, Miguel Alvarez, Bobbie Andelson, Diane Anderson, Ian E. Anderson, Tomika Anderson, Roshun Andrews, Walter Armstrong, James Lee Aronson, Mark Aurigemma, Marjorie Backman, Erin Baer, Andrew Bagnall, Elysia Bandog, Bob Barnett, Mike Barr, Marge Barton, Brooks Bebon, Timothy Beemer, Tom Beer, LD Beghtol, Eli Belil, Lapo Belmestieri, Todd Bender, Alec Bentley, Elliot Bishow, Gary Blunt, Phil Geoffrey Bond, Phillip Bond, Marvelyn Brown, Stephan Buckingham, Shaun Burger, Nick Burns, Laura Burton, Ryan Canty, David Capogna, Brian Carden, Scott-Lee Cash, Kareema Charles, Sally Chew, Erich Chu, Stephen Cloutier, Greg Concha, Bob Cook, Sara Coppin, Dennis Corbett, Amber Cortes, Muriel Crane-Rosenblum, Pedro Cruz, Anthony Curatolo, Paul Daily, James Dale, Dennis C. Daniel, Kimberlyn David, Casey Davidson, Gregory Dean, Gamalier De Jesus, Rafael DeJesus, Robert Del Deo, Kathy DeLeon, Michelle Delio, Mark De Solla Price, Coleen De Vol, Kevin Doherty, Kevin C. Donahue, Steve Doppelt, Tom Doyle, David Drake, Steven Duarte, Keith Dupont, Marisa Dussel, Stefani Eads, Shanita Ealey, Johnjon Emigh, Christian Evans, David Evans, Greg Evans, Forest Evashevski, Stephanie Fairyington, Kenyon Farrow, Emmy Favilla, Kate Ferguson, Cindra Feuer, Belinda Filippelli, B. Scott Finley, Nick Fowler, Willette Francis, Keisha Franklin, Vincent Gagliostro, Meave Gallagher, Molly Gallagher, Cassidy Gardner, Jonathan Gaskell, Kathleen Gates, Linda Gates, David Geller, David Gelman, Stephen Gendin, Steven Giacona, Jennifer Gong, Angel Gonzalez, Cristina González, Cameron Gorman, Dana Gornitzki, Jeremy Grayzel, Alicia Green, Shavon S. Greene, Joel Griffiths, Will Guilliams, Alexis Gumby, Oriol R. Gutierrez Jr., Brittany Hall, Mitchell Hall, Michael Halliday, Casey Halter, Lauren Hauptman, Timothy Healea, India Hearn, Bill Henning, Regan Hofmann, Jillian Holness, Jeff Hoover, Gabrielle Horn, Tim Horn, Tonia Howick, Jennifer Hsu, Clara Huang, Bob Ickes, Andrej Jechropov, Dorshia Johnson, LaToya Johnson, Daniel L. Johnston, Brent Jordheim, Hillary Joseph, Nicole Joseph, Comfort Nnana Kalu, Michelle Kaminer, Esther Kaplan, Joel Kaplan, Jonathan Jacob Kaplan, Tony Karon, Lida Marie Keene, Doriot Kim, Karl Klippel, Elsie Kmech, Geoffrey Knox, Fred Kostbar, Eugenio Kovacs, Shana Naomi Krochmal, John La, Annie Lai, Lark Lands, Alicia S. Lara, Bryan Lara, Kent M.C. Lau, Bob Lederer, John Lee, Paul Lee, Randall Leers, Brendan Lemon, Ken Letavish, Susan Mary Levey, Matthew Levine, David Levinson, Arnie Lewis, Mark Leydorf, Celeste Lodevole, Pam Long, Karen Lopienski, Jesse Heiwa Loving, Greg Lugliani, Phoebe Mackay, Manjula Martin, Suzy Martin, Steven Martinez, Akiko Matsuda, Winnie McCroy, Shari McKoy, Kabrina McLaughlin, Joe Mejía, Kenneth Mercado, Kenny Miles, Eric Minton, Jason Mischka, Carlos Moore, Anthony Morales, Xavier Morales, Al Morris, Paul W. Morris, Steve Morrison, Jennifer Morton, Valarie Mulero, Ben Munisteri, Timothy Murphy, Amanda Myers, Marlo Ned, Kat Noel, Chris Nutter, Doris O'Donnell, Nicole Oetama, Ned O'Gorman, Kevin O'Leary, Janet Oliver, Nicholas Olson, Karen Pantelides, Brad Peebles, Robert T. Pelham, Leticia Perea, Richard Pérez-Feria, Lawrence D. Peters, Gary Petonke, Christopher Petrikin, Will Plummer, Lori Pollicino, Michael Polson, Steven M. Price, RonniLyn Pustil, Marianne Quirk, Caroline Rabiecki, Greg Rabiecki, Angelo Ragaza, Chris Reeves, Kathleen Reeves, Michael Richman, Elida Rivera, Victor Rivera, Yuvi Rivera, Mark Robinson, Jeff Roeske, Yesenia Robles, Benjamin Ryan, Philip Salvatore, Christie Leigh Scanlan, Dick Scanlan, Diana Scholl, Joy Scopa, Henry Scott, Lucile Scott, Bart Senior, Christina Sharpe, Aiden Shaw, Ed Shaw, Karen Sherman, Juliana Shulman, Louise Sloan, George Slowik Jr., Michael Solita, Regan Solmo, Josh Sparber, Trey Speegle, Jason Spitzer, Peter Staley, Adam Stiles, Trent Straube, Megan Strub, Sean O'Brien Strub, J.C. Suarès, Sandrea-Lee Swaby, Michelle Tan, Kellee Terrell, David Thomas, John Thompson, David Thorpe, Anika Tillery, David Tinmouth, Elliot Torres, John Patrick Trant, Harry Trantham, Jerry Tuccillo, Lauren Tuck, Johnny Valentin, Cathryn Vandewater, Giovanni Vitacolonna, Reed Vreeland, Scott Wald, Christine Weigel, Geoffrey Weiss, Pamela Weis, Kendall Wenaas, Ryan Westbrook, Laura Whitehorn, LeRoy Whitfield, Lauren Wiezorek, Joseph Wilbeck, Dennis Williams, Kayreth Williams, Scott Williams, Phill Wilson, Christopher Wiss, Tiffany Wolf, James Wortman, Paraskevi Xenophontos, Alison Zack, Danielle Zielinski, Max Zimbert, Ross Zuckerman, Ian Zund, Melanie Zurlo

A special thanks to three pets honored on past POZ mastheads: Olive, Willy and Zoom

www.ingramcontent.com/pod-product-compliance
Lightning Source LLC
Chambersburg PA
CBHW060801270326
41926CB00002B/55